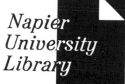

# SYSTEMATIC REVIEWS

# SYSTEMATIC REVIEWS

Edited by

**IAIN CHALMERS**
*Director, UK Cochrane Centre*
*NHS Research and Development Programme,*
*Oxford*

and

**DOUGLAS G ALTMAN**
*Head, Medical Statistics Laboratory,*
*Imperial Cancer Research Fund, London*

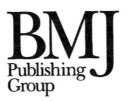

BMJ
Publishing
Group

*This book is dedicated to*

## Thomas C Chalmers

*in appreciation of his many pioneering contributions to the science of reviewing health research, and in particular, for the first clear demonstration of the dangers of relying on traditional reviews of research to guide clinical practice.*

The picture of Maastricht Carnivalists (p 12) is reproduced with permission from Simson of Barnaby's.

© BMJ Publishing Group 1995

Iain Chalmers's work is © Crown copyright 1995

First published in 1995
Reprinted September 1995
by the BMJ Publishing Group, BMA House, Tavistock Square,
London WC1H 9JR

**British Library Cataloguing in Publication Data**

A catalogue record for this book is available
from the British Library

ISBN 0-7279-0904-5

Typeset in Great Britain by Apek Typesetters Ltd., Nailsea, Bristol
Printed and bound in Great Britain by Latimer Trend & Company Ltd, Plymouth

# Contents

CONTENTS

# Foreword

Reviews of the results of research have become essential for anyone who is serious about trying to cope with ever-increasing tidal waves of new research evidence. Wider recognition of the key role of reviews in synthesising the results of primary research has prompted people to consider the validity of reviews. Unfortunately, it is usually not possible to judge whether conventional narrative reviews are trustworthy. In contrast to reports of primary research, such reviews rarely make explicit their objectives, materials, and methods. In the 1970s psychologists drew attention to the systematic steps needed to minimise biases and random errors in reviews of research. It was not until 1987 that Mulrow first drew attention to the poor scientific quality of reviews of clinical research.[1] The following year Oxman and Guyatt published guidelines to help readers assess the quality of reviews in health care.[2]

In an applied field of research such as the evaluation of health care, reviews which have been prepared with disregard for scientific principles can have serious consequences. In 1992, after presenting a landmark comparison of what was being recommended in textbooks of cardiology and what could have been known if their authors had applied scientific principles to their task, Antman and his colleagues noted that "because reviewers have not used scientific methods, advice on some lifesaving therapies has been delayed for more than a decade, while other treatments have been recommended long after controlled research has shown them to be harmful."[3]

It was because of a recognition that this worrying state of affairs needed greater exposure and discussion, that the BMJ and the UK Cochrane Centre collaborated in organising a meeting in London in July 1993 to discuss aspects of the science of reviewing clinical research. The chapters in this book are based on papers presented at that meeting, which were published in earlier versions in the

BMJ during 1994. The first two - by Cynthia Mulrow, and by Paul Knipschild - introduce and illustrate systematic reviews. Kay Dickersin, Roberta Scherer and Carol Lefebvre, and Michael Clarke and Lesley Stewart discuss the data collection challenges confronting those preparing systematic reviews. Simon Thompson and Hans Eysenck concentrate on quantitative synthesis of primary data to yield an overall summary statistic (meta-analysis). These chapters make it clear that interpretation of the summary statistics generated through meta-analysis will often present challenges, particularly when the primary data have not been derived from controlled experiments. In the penultimate chapter Andrew Oxman provides guidelines for assessing reviews; and finally one of us (IC) and Brian Haynes describe how systematic reviews are being prepared, updated, and disseminated by the international network of people who together constitute the Cochrane Collaboration. Because the chapters do not offer comprehensive coverage of the field, the book concludes with a methodological bibliography of further reading. For those wishing to explore the science of reviewing research in greater depth we hope that this bibliography will satisfy the appetite that the book is intended to stimulate.

A word about terminology: both the 1993 meeting and the book based on the proceedings have very deliberately used the term "systematic review" rather than some of the alternatives which are in use. Use of this term implies only that a review has been prepared using some kind of systematic approach to minimising biases and random errors, and that the components of the approach will be documented in a materials and methods section. Other terms, particularly "meta-analysis," have caused confusion because of the implication that a systematic approach to reviews *must* entail quantitative synthesis of primary data to yield an overall summary statistic (meta-analysis). As we hope this book will help to make clear, this is not the case. In addition to those circumstances in which statistical synthesis of results of primary research is not advisable, there will be others in which it is quite simply impossible. It is just as important to take steps to control biases in reviews in these circumstances as it is to do so in circumstances in which meta-analysis is both indicated and possible.

Iain Chalmers
Doug Altman
December 1994

1 Mulrow CD. The medical review article: state of the science. *Ann Intern Med* 1987; **106**: 485-8.
2 Oxman AD, Guyatt GH. Guidelines for reading literature reviews. *Can Med Assoc J* 1988; **138**: 697-703.
3 Antman EM, Lau J, Kupelnick B, Mosteller F, Chalmers TC. A comparison of results of meta-analyses and randomized control trials and recommendations of clinical experts. *JAMA* 1992; **268**: 240-8.

# Biographical notes

Iain Chalmers was director of the National Perinatal Epidemiology Unit between 1978 and 1992, when he became director of the UK Cochrane Centre in Oxford. The UK Cochrane Centre, which was established to support the Research and Development Programme of the British National Health Service, is one of an increasing number of Cochrane centres helping to coordinate the Cochrane Collaboration - a rapidly growing international network of individuals preparing, maintaining, and disseminating systematic reviews of research on the effects of health care.

Douglas G Altman is head of the Medical Statistics Laboratory at the Imperial Cancer Research Fund in London. His many research interests include the use and abuse of statistics in medical journals, models for prognosis, and studies of medical measurement. He previously worked at St Thomas's Hospital Medical School, and spent 11 years at the MRC Clinical Research Centre at Northwick Park, where he worked in a wide variety of medical areas. He is author of *Practical Statistics for Medical Research* (1991), coauthor of *Statistics in Practice* (1982), and coeditor of *Statistics with Confidence* (1989).

# 1 Rationale for systematic reviews

CYNTHIA D MULROW

## Summary

Systematic reviews of research evidence are invaluable scientific activities. The rationale for such reviews is well established. Health care providers, researchers, and policy makers are inundated with unmanageable amounts of information; they need systematic reviews to efficiently integrate existing information and provide data for rational decision making. Systematic reviews establish whether scientific findings are consistent and can be generalised across populations, settings, and treatment variations, or whether findings vary significantly by particular subsets. Explicit methods used in systematic reviews limit bias and will improve reliability and accuracy of conclusions. Meta-analysis can increase power and precision of estimates of treatment effects and exposure risks.

Systematic review of research evidence is a fundamental scientific activity. Its rationale is grounded firmly in several premises. Firstly, large quantities of information must be reduced into palatable pieces for digestion. Over two million articles are published annually in the biomedical literature in over 20 000 journals—literally a small mountain of information. For example, about 4400 pages were devoted to approximately 1100 articles in the *BMJ* and *New England Journal of Medicine*, combined, in 1992. In a stack, two million such articles would rise 500 m.

1

Clearly, systematic review is needed to refine these unmanageable amounts of information. Through critical exploration, evaluation, and synthesis the systematic review separates the insignificant, unsound, or redundant deadwood from the salient and critical studies that are worthy of reflection.[2]

Secondly, various decision makers need to integrate the critical pieces of available biomedical information. Systematic reviews are used by more specialised integrators, such as economic and decision analysts, to estimate the variables and outcomes that are included in their evaluations. Both systematic and more specialised integrations are used by clinicians to keep abreast of the primary research in a given field as well as to remain literate in broader aspects of medicine.[3, 4] Researchers use the review to identify, justify, and refine hypotheses; recognise and avoid pitfalls of previous work; estimate sample sizes; and delineate important ancillary or adverse effects and covariates that warrant consideration in future studies. Finally, health policy makers use systematic reviews to formulate guidelines and legislation concerning the use of certain diagnostic tests and treatment strategies.

## An efficient scientific technique

Thirdly, the systematic review is an efficient scientific technique. Although sometimes arduous and time consuming, a review is usually quicker and less costly than embarking on a new study. Just as important, a review can prevent meandering down an already explored path. Continuously updated reviews, as exemplified by the *Cochrane Database of Systematic Reviews*,[5] can shorten the time between medical research discoveries and clinical implementation of effective diagnostic or treatment strategies. A landmark example of cumulative meta-analyses and its benefits is shown in figure 1·1 which gives odds ratios and 95% confidence intervals for 33 trials that compared intravenous streptokinase with a placebo or no therapy in patients who had been hospitalised for acute myocardial infarctions. The left side of the figure shows that the effect of treatment with streptokinase on mortality was favourable in 25 of the 33 trials, but in only six was statistical significance achieved. The overall pooled estimate of treatment effect given at the bottom significantly favoured treatment. The right side of the figure shows the same data presented as if a new or cumulative meta-analysis was performed each time the results of a new trial were reported. The years during which the

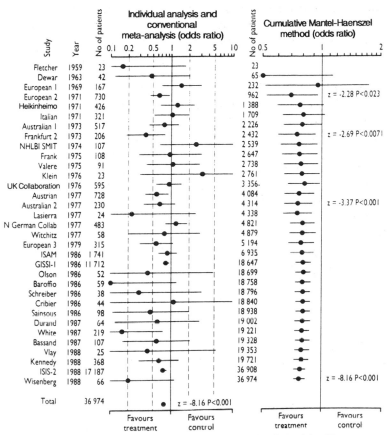

Figure 1.1 Conventional and cumulative meta-analysis of 33 trials of intravenous streptokinase for acute myocardial infarction. Odds ratios and 95% confidence intervals for effect of treatment on mortality are shown on a logarithmic scale[6]

treatment effect became statistically significant were 1971 for a two sided P value of < 0·05, 1973 for a P value of 0·01, and 1977 for a P value of < 0·001. This cumulative type of systematic review indicated that intravenous streptokinase could have been shown to be life saving almost 20 years ago, long before its submission to and approval by the United States Food and Drug Administration and its general promotion in practice.

*Generalisability, consistency—and inconsistency*

Fourthly, the generalisability of scientific findings can be established in systematic reviews. The diversity of multiple

3

reviewed studies provides an interpretive context not available in any one study.[7] This is because studies addressing similar questions often use different eligibility criteria for participants, different definitions of disease, different methods of measuring or defining exposure, different variations of a treatment, and different study designs.[8]

Closely related to generalisability, a fifth reason for systematic reviews is to assess the consistency of relationships. Assessments of whether effects are in the same directions and of the same general magnitudes, given the variation in study protocols, can be made. More specifically, systematic reviews can assess consistency among studies of the same intervention or even among studies of different interventions (for example, varying doses or intensities or classes of therapeutic agents).[9] Consistency of treatment effects across different diseases with common underlying pathophysiology and consistency of risk factors across study populations can be ascertained.

Conversely, a sixth reason for systematic reviews is to explain data inconsistencies and conflicts in data. Whether a treatment strategy is effective in one setting and not in another or among some patients and not others can be assessed. Furthermore, whether findings from a single study stand alone for any reason such as uniqueness of study population, study quality, or outcome measure can be explored.

## Power and precision

Seventhly, an often cited advantage of quantitative systematic reviews in particular is increased power. Quantitative reviews or meta-analysis have been likened to "a tower of statistical power that allows researchers to rise above the body of evidence, survey the landscape, and map out future directions."[10] An example of meta-analysis improving statistical power is shown in the Cochrane Collaboration's logo (figure 1·2) (see chapter 8), which depicts the results of seven trials that evaluated the effects of a short course of corticosteroids given to women expected to give birth prematurely. Only two trials had clear cut, statistically significant effects; but when data from all of the studies were pooled, the "sample size" (and thus power) increased. This yielded a definitive significant combined effect estimate which indicated strongly that corticosteroids reduce the risk of babies dying from complications of immaturity. The advantage of

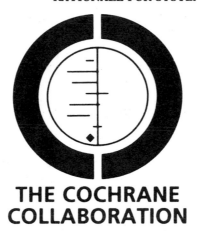

## THE COCHRANE
## COLLABORATION

Figure 1.2 The Cochrane Collaboration logo shows how pooling data reveals the significance of treatment effects

increasing power is particularly relevant to conditions of relatively low event rates or when small effects are being assessed.

Eighthly, quantitative systematic reviews allow increased precision in estimates of effect. On the right side of figure 1 the cumulative meta-analysis shows that increasing sample size from temporally consecutive studies resulted in continued narrowing of confidence intervals even though efficacy had been established in the early 1970s.[6] Particularly noteworthy, two very large trials— the 1986 study of the Gruppo Italiano per lo Studio della Streptochinasi nell'Infarto Miocardico (GISSI) involving 11 712 patients and the 1988 second international study of infarct survival (ISIS-2) involving 17 187 patients did not change the already established evidence of efficacy though they increased precision by narrowing the confidence intervals slightly.

*Accurate assessment*

A final rationale for systematic reviews is accuracy, or at least an improved reflection of reality. Traditional reviews have been criticised as haphazard and biased, subject to the idiosyncratic impressions of the individual reviewer.[11] Systematic reviews and meta-analyses apply explicit scientific principles aimed at reducing random and systematic errors.[12] Whether such reviews will lead to greater reliability, and by inference greater accuracy, has not yet been established clearly.[8]

5

At the very least, the use of explicit methods allows assessment of what was done and thus increases the ability to replicate results or understanding of why results and conclusions of some reviews differ. In addition, reviewers using traditional methods are less likely to detect small but signficant effects than are reviewers using formal systematic and statistical techniques.[13] Finally, traditional review recommendations lag behind and sometimes vary significantly from continuously updated or cumulative meta-analyses.[14] Figure 1.3 shows that pooled data from 15 randomised trials published before 1990 found no evidence of mortality

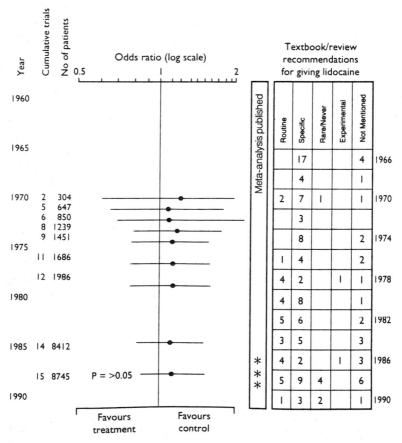

Figure 1.3 Cumulative meta-analysis by year of publication or randomised controlled trials of prophylactic lidocaine for acute myocardial infarction, and recommendations of clinical expert reviewers (adapted from Antman *et al*[14])

benefit associated with prophylactic lidocaine for acute myocardial infarction. Despite this evidence, most pertinent traditional reviews continued to recommend prophylactic lidocaine. Antman *et al* have shown also that many effective treatments for reducing mortality due to acute myocardial infarction are not being recommended as often as they might be.[6][14]

*Summary*

There is a myriad of reasons to herald systematic reviews, including meta-analyses. The hundreds of hours spent conducting a scientific study ultimately contribute only one piece of an enormous puzzle. The value of any single study is derived from how it fits with and expands previous work, as well as from the study's intrinsic properties.[15] Through systematic review the puzzle's intricacies may be disentangled.

The vast amount of available information underscores the value of systematic reviews. As T S Eliot asked in his poem "The Rock," "Where is the knowledge we have lost in information?" Decision makers of various types are inundated with unmanageable amounts of information. They have great need for systematic reviews that separate the known from the unknown and that save them from the position of knowing less than has been proved.[16]

Advantages of the systematic review are many. Whether scientific findings are consistent and can be generalised across populations, settings, and treatment variations or whether findings vary significantly by particular subsets can be gleaned. Unique advantages of quantitative systematic reviews (meta-analyses) are increased power and precision in estimating effects and risks. Both qualitative and quantitative systematic reviews, with their explicit methods, will limit bias and improve the reliability and accuracy of recommendations.

I thank Dr Rosalva M Solis for her assistance in the preparation of this chapter.

# References

1 Ad Hoc Working Group for Critical Appraisal of the Medical Literature. Academia and clinic: a proposal for more informative abstracts of clinical articles. *Ann Intern Med* 1987; **106**: 598–604.
2 Morgan PP. Review articles. 2. The literature jungle. *Can Med Assoc J* 1986; **134**: 98–9.
3 Garfield E. Reviewing review literature. Part 2. The place of reviews in the scientific literature. *Current Contents* 1987; **30**: 3–5.

4 Lederberg J. Introduction. *Annual Review of Computer Science* 1986; **1**: 5–9.
5 *Cochrane Collaboration*. *Cochrane Database of Systematic Reviews*. *Disc issue 1*. London: BMJ Publishing Group/Update Software, 1995.
6 Lau J, Antman EM, Jimenez-Silva J, Kupelnick B, Mosteller F, Chalmers TC. Cumulative meta-analysis of therapeutic trials for myocardial infarction. *N Engl J Med* 1992; **327**: 248–54.
7 Light RJ, Pillemer DB. *Summing up: the science of reviewing research*. Cambridge: MA: Harvard University Press, 1984.
8 Dickersin K, Berlin JA. Meta-analysis: state-of-the-science. *Epidemiol Rev* 1992; **14**: 154–76.
9 Boissel JP, Blanchard J, Panak E, Peyrieux JC, Sacks H. Considerations for the meta-analysis of randomized clinical trials. *Controlled Clin Trials* 1989; **10**: 254–81.
10 Gelber RD, Goldhirsch A. Meta-analysis: the fashion of summing-up evidence. *Ann Oncol* 1991; **2**: 461–8.
11 Mulrow CD. The medical review article: state of the science. *Ann Intern Med* 1987; **106**: 485–8.
12 Oxman AD, Guyatt GH. Guidelines for reading literature reviews. *Can Med Assoc J* 1988; **138**: 697–703.
13 Cooper HM, Rosenthal R. Statistical versus traditional procedures for summarizing research findings. *Psychol Bull* 1980; **87**: 442–9.
14 Antman EM, Lau J, Kupelnick B, Mosteller F, Chalmers TC. A comparison of results of meta-analyses of randomized control trials and recommendations of clinical experts. *JAMA* 1992; **268**: 240–8.
15 Cooper HM. *The integrative research review: a systematic approach*. Beverley Hills, CA: Sage Publications, 1984.
16 Glass GV. Primary, secondary, and meta-analysis of research. *Educational Researcher* 1976; **5**: 3–8.

# 2 Some examples of systematic reviews

PAUL KNIPSCHILD

## Summary

Reviewing research evidence is a scientific inquiry that needs a clear design to preclude bias. It is a real enterprise if one aims at completeness of the evidence on a certain subject. Going through refereed English language journals is not enough. On line databases are helpful, but mainly as a starting point. This article gives examples of systematic reviews on vitamin C for the common cold, pyridoxine for the premenstrual syndrome, homoeopathy, and physiotherapy.

You will have heard of Maastricht—in 1992 the European Union treaty was signed there. Some people dislike Maastricht because it seems to stand for the ideal of the United States of Europe, but many of us in Maastricht do not even know what the treaty is about. What we like is to sit together and enjoy our Burgundian way of living. Maastricht is one big sidewalk café.

People in my town are very inventive in finding reasons for painting the town red. Of the many festivals that we have, carnival in the late winter is definitely number one. Anyone born and bred in Maastricht would not dream of escaping the noise, the jigging, and the many beers. For almost a week we live in sin and after that we are so depleted that we need a few days off to recover. Nearly every good carnivalist gets a sore throat, a stuffy nose, and other signs of a common cold: it is a marker that we have done our duty.

## A carnival trial?

Some years ago a doctor who was not from Maastricht asked me to help set up a preventive trial on vitamin C and the common cold. I immediately thought of making it a carnival trial. So I suggested, "Take 200 carnivalists and randomise them to placebo or vitamin C before the carnival storm breaks. You will have the answer right away."

But then I had to think more professionally. "Wait a minute," I said, "did you review the literature first?" I explained to him that it was wrong to begin a new trial if you have not done a thorough search for existing evidence. Off he went, but he was back a week later. "Did you know," he started, "that double Nobel laureate Linus Pauling never has a common cold because he marinates himself in vitamin C?" I told my visitor that case reports could not convince me anymore. "It is trials that I want," I added, "trials and nothing less."

## Example of a non-systematic review

Then my visitor showed me Pauling's 1986 book, *How to Live Longer and Feel Better*.[1] "Here it is," he said, "chapter 13 tells you all you want to know about trials of vitamin C and the common cold: Pauling refers to more than 30 to prove his point. And nearly all are positive."

The chapter in the book was an updated version of Pauling's earlier bestseller, *Vitamin C and the Common Cold*. It is a good example of an extensive but non-systematic review of the literature. It does not tell the reader anything about the design of his survey of trials. For a start, what were the admission criteria for his studies and where did he look for them? Was the methodological quality assessed blindly, or at least independently of the outcome? And how did Pauling decide whether the result of a certain trial, and the combined result of the better ones was positive, negative, or in between?

The hazard of a haphazard review is obvious. Probably all of us are prejudiced and tend to focus on what we like to see. And, even worse, some tend to dismiss anything that does not suit their purpose. This makes it worthwhile to set certain rules before starting a review process. Reviews are scientific inquiries and they need a clear design to preclude bias.

## An exhaustive search

Some colleagues and I, wanting to outsmart Pauling and his supporters, made a plan and started a new and exhaustive search.[2] Of course this included Medline from 1966 up to 1991. Our literature computer cranked out lots of studies, among them 22 controlled trials. Next we started checking the references in these articles. The first check yielded 15 additional trials. Then we checked the references of the references, which yielded another nine. The third check gave us only one extra, bringing the total to 47. (If you do the same with Embase you find $15 + 16 + 11 + 2 = 44$ trials, all which you have already found with Medline and the three checks of references.)

What happens if you still do not stop there? We went on searching *Index Medicus* from 1940 to 1965 manually, checked through *Current Contents*, bent over textbooks on vitamins (including Pauling's book), wrote and talked to researchers who had done interesting trials, went to special libraries such as Hoffman La Roche's "World of Vitamins" in Switzerland, and told everyone that we were after vitamin C and the common cold. By doing this we added another 14 trials, bringing our total to 61.

We feel that our collection is still far from complete. With the Medline search we got only 36% of the studies, but checking the references, and the references of the references was very rewarding: this provided 75%. Only fanatical collectors can do much better.

Next we graded every trial according to its methodological soundness, independently of the results, of course.[3] On a scale from 0 to 12, 15 of the 61 trials scored seven or more points. Interestingly, only one of these 15 trials was not in Medline.

## Vitamin C for your cold?

To know what vitamin C can do to a common cold, you should of course rely heavily on the results of the best studies. It does not make sense to combine the top 15 with the other 46 and then do a meta-analysis. Meta-analysis is also inappropriate if there are large differences between trials in the choice of patients, interventions, and measurements of effect.

After a review of the literature,[3] [4] here is my conclusion: vitamin C, even in gram quantities per day, cannot prevent a cold. On the other hand, if you already have a cold, a megadose of, say

11

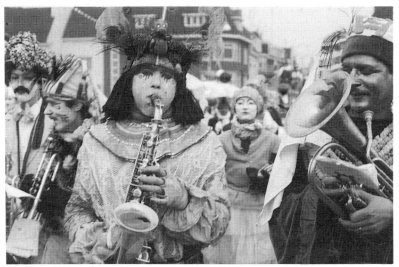

After carnival week, colds are common in Maastricht's residents as they recover—
the perfect testing ground for effects of vitamin C

1 g vitamin C may slightly decrease the duration and severity of your cold (perhaps by 10%).

What about Pauling's review? He did not mention five of our top 15 studies (all published before 1986), and two others were referred to only in passing. The other eight trials were discussed in his book, but some could not show a preventive effect because they considered only the possible therapeutic benefit of vitamin C. Two preventive trials that failed to detect any effect were "unfortunately flawed," according to Pauling. Yet, if you read his colourful story instead of a rather dull systematic review, it all sounds very convincing. He ends his case: "Catching a cold and letting it run its course is a sign that you are not taking enough vitamin C."

Pauling also emphasises an important side effect of taking a megadose of vitamin C (and other nutrients) every day. He believes that, if you do this, together with a few other healthful practices, from youth or middle age, you can "extend your life and years of wellbeing by 25 or even 35 years."

*New trial*

If you want to do a new trial, there are at least two reasons why you should do a systematic review first. One reason is that you can learn a lot from earlier studies. Talking to the authors of earlier studies is especially useful; it should be part of the preparation for a new trial. They will tell you about things that went wrong but cannot be found in their papers. It prevents you from making the same mistakes.

The other reason for a review is that sometimes a new trial can add little to what is already known. Never believe beforehand that you are the first to study a certain subject. Many honest investigators missed earlier research or at least did not refer to it in their publications. Here is one example.

Some patients, and doctors for that matter,[5] believe that pyridoxine (vitamin B-6) helps in the premenstrual syndrome. What does the literature say? Researchers from Oxford published a trial on this subject in 1989, referring to five earlier trials.[6] By then I knew of six other trials (including two on premenstrual mastalgia), of which two were large, well performed trials. One year later, researchers from Philadelphia also published a report on pyridoxine and the premenstrual syndrome.[7] They did not refer to nine of the 12 trials published before 1990, which included four well performed trials.[8]

Would these researchers have started their studies if they had known of all other published and ongoing trials? Every important trial that they had missed showed an ambiguous or frankly unpromising result.

### Foreign languages

Good reviewers should know their languages, or at least have people around who are not afraid of reading "Eine Placebo-kontrolierte Doppel-blindstudie" or "Une étude randomisée à double insu face au placebo." There is nothing fundamentally wrong with publications in "foreign" langauges. Some papers are of high quality, but the authors are not yet familiar with the idea of writing a report for one of the well known English language journals.

### Grey literature

There is much grey literature around. Of course you must include publications in less famous, non-refereed journals (and even "internal" reports) in your systematic review[9]—you are the referee.

I recently discussed the importance of searching the grey literature on alternative medicine.[10] It is a real enterprise that takes its toll ih blood, sweat, and tears. One of the examples I gave was homoeopathy.

Helped by alternative researchers, my colleagues and I turned many libraries upside down to get a collection of 107 controlled trials (published before May 1991). Medline yielded only 18 publications. Checking the references and the references of the references increased the number to 30, still not more than 28%. For homoeopathy, other sources such as congress reports and dissertations (from Germany and France) were more fruitful.[2]

Most (61%) of the trials that we could find on homoeopathy were published in languages other than English. We graded all trials for their methodological quality on a scale of 0 to 100; 16 scored 60 or more points. Only three of the better (full) publications were in English.[11]


## The physiotherapy literature

Several years ago my department began to study physiotherapy. For dubious reasons the Dutch government considered classical physiotherapy to be mainstream and manual therapy to be alternative medicine. In our trial manual therapy seemed more effective for patients with persistent spine problems.[12]

We started, however, with searching the literature.[13] It really got out of control, partly because further trials on back pain, shoulder stiffness, and ankle sprains were also initiated. In the end we asked everybody to help us find controlled trials on exercise therapy, manipulation, or physical applications. Of course we searched Medline and Embase, but we also glanced at many unindexed journals, books, and congress reports. And we checked references endlessly.

So far we have found about 750 randomised clinical trials (and another 750 controlled studies without random allocation). Most were done among patients with back pain (175), knee problems (114), lung dysfunction (77), shoulder stiffness (51), stroke (45), and ankle problems (43). Trials have been published in almost every journal that you can think of. Again, many of the trials that we found were not in Medline or Embase. An unindexed journal called *Physiotherapy* was second (with 23 trials) after *Archives of Physical Medicine and Rehabilitation* (38 trials). Half of all trials were published in English, but this proportion may decrease now that we are trying harder to find publications in other languages.

As the trials come in, a special group grades the studies blindly according to their methodological quality. Unfortunately, the quality seems to be low. On a scale from 0 to 100 the median is only 40, and only 2% of the trials score 60 points or more. I am well aware that efficacy studies on physiotherapy are more difficult than on drugs, but one can do much better. To improve clinical research on physiotherapy my university has started a special doctoral programme for physiotherapists who are interested in a research career.

### Summing up

I have presented several examples of reviews. The first was on vitamin C and the common cold, for which there is already a megadose of literature. One extensive but non-systematic review seems to be seriously biased towards the ideas of the author. The example also shows that searching with Medline yields only a limited number of publications. However, checking the references, and the references of the references, is very rewarding.

One of my examples was about pyridoxine in the treatment of patients with premenstrual syndrome. I wondered whether the researchers of recently published trials would have started their studies if they had known of all published or ongoing trials. Next I argued, using homoeopathy as an example, that good researchers do not restrict their reviews to refereed papers, or papers that are written in English. It takes less time and money to translate a paper than to do a new trial.

Finally I told you about our large collection of trials on physiotherapy. Of course, we also use them to write reviews on physiotherapeutic topics. The *BMJ* published some of them, showing its interest in systematic reviews.[14 15] The Cochrane Collaboration (see chapter 8) has invited my colleagues and me to help with its enormous enterprise to have every old and new trial computerised—we will be glad to do that for physiotherapy.

Ideally, information on all published and ongoing research on a certain subject should be indexed and made widely accessible. Such a dynamic vade mecum, which should be checked by every investigator who thinks of doing a clinical trial, is needed; so the Cochrane Collaboration deserves all the support it can get.

## SOME EXAMPLES OF SYSTEMATIC REVIEWS

I thank the many people in the Department of Epidemiology, University of Limburg, who actually spent more time searching the literature than I did. The project was supported by several grants of the Dutch Ministry of Welfare, Public Health, and Cultural Affairs.

1 Pauling L. *How to live longer and feel better.* New York: Freeman, 1986
2 Kleijnen J, Knipschild P. The comprehensiveness of Medline and Embase computer searches. Searches for controlled trials of homoeopathy, ascorbic acid for common cold and ginkgo biloba for cerebral insufficiency and intermittant claudication. *Pharm Weekbl [Sci]* 1992; **14**: 316–20.
3 Kleijnen J, ter Riet G, Knipschild P. Vitamin C and the common cold; review of a megadose of literature. In: Kleijnen J. Food supplements and their efficacy [dissertation]. Maastricht, University of Limburg, 1991.
4 Hemilä H. Vitamin C and the common cold. *Br J Nutr* 1992; **67**: 3–16.
5 Knipschild P, Kleijnen J, ter Riet G. Belief in the efficacy of alternative medicine among general practitioners in the Netherlands. *Soc Sci Med* 1990; **31**: 625–6.
6 Doll H, Brown S, Thurston A, Vessey M. Pyridoxine (vitamin $B_6$) and the premenstrual syndrome: a randomised crossover trial. *JR Coll Gen Pract* 1989; **39**: 364–8.
7 Krutan Berman M, Taylor ML, Freeman E. Vitamin B–6 in premenstrual syndrome. *J Am Diet Assoc* 1990; **90**: 859–61.
8 Kleijnen J, ter Riet G, Knipschild P. Vitamin B6 in the treatment of the premenstrual syndrome—a review. *Br J Obstet Gynaecol* 1990; **97**: 847–52.
9 Cook DJ, Guyatt GH, Ryan G, Clifton J, Buckingham L, Willan A, *et al.* Should unpublished data be included in meta-analyses? Current convictions and controversies. *JAMA* 1993; **269**: 2749–53.
10 Knipschild P. Searching for alternatives: loser pays. *Lancet* 1993; **341**: 1135–6.
11 Kleijnen J, Knipschild P, ter Riet G. Clinical trials of homoeopathy. *BMJ* 1991; **302**: 316–23.
12 Koes BW, Bouter LM, van Mameren H, Essers AHM, Verstegen GMJR, *et al.* Randomised clinical trial of manual therapy and physiotherapy for persistent back and neck complaints. Results of one year follow-up. *BMJ* 1992; **304**:601–5.
13 Beckerman H, Bouter L, eds. Effectiviteit van fysiotherapie. Een literatuuronderzoek. Maastricht, Limburg: University of Limburg, Department of Epidemiology and Biostatistics, 1991.
14 Koes BW, Assendelft WJJ, van der Heijden GJMG, Bouter LM, Knipschild PG. Spinal manipulation and mobilization for back and neck pain. A blinded review. *BMJ* 1991; **303**: 1298–303.
15 Koes BW, Bouter LM, Beckerman H, van der Heijden GJMG, Knipschild PG. Physiotherapy exercises and back pain. A blinded review. *BMJ* 1991; **302**: 1572–6.

# 3 Identifying relevant studies for systematic reviews

KAY DICKERSIN, ROBERTA SCHERER,
CAROL LEFEBVRE

## Summary

*Objective*—To examine the sensitivity and precision of Medline searching for randomised clinical trials.

*Design*—(i) comparison of results of Medline searches to a "gold standard" of known randomised clinical trials in ophthalmology published in 1988; (ii) systematic review (meta-analysis) of results of similar, but separate, studies from many fields of medicine.

*Populations*—Randomised clinical trials published in 1988 in journals indexed in Medline, and those not indexed in Medline and identified by hand search, comprised the gold standard. Gold standards for the other studies combined in the meta-analysis were based on: randomised clinical trials published in any journal, whether indexed in Medline or not; those published in any journal indexed in Medline; or those published in a selected group of journals indexed in Medline.

*Main outcome measures*—Sensitivity (proportion of the total number of known randomised clinical trials identified by the search) and precision (proportion of publications retrieved by Medline that were actually randomised clinical trials) were calculated for each study and combined to obtain weighted means. Searches producing the "best" sensitivity were used for sensitivity and precision estimates when multiple searches were performed.

*Results*—The sensitivity of searching for ophthalmology randomised clinical trials published in 1988 was 82%, when the gold standard was for any journal, 87% for any journal indexed in Medline, and 88% for selected journals indexed in Medline. Weighted means for sensitivity across all studies were 51%, 77% and 63%, respectively. The weighted mean for precision was 9% (median 33%). Most searchers seemed not to use freetext subject terms and truncation of those terms.

*Conclusion*—Although the indexing terms available for searching Medline for randomised clinical trials have improved, sensitivity still remains unsatisfactory. A mechanism is needed to register known trials, preferably by retrospective tagging of Medline entries, and incorporating trials published before 1966 and in journals not indexed by Medline into the system.

## Background

Thorough data collection is of primary importance in preparing a systematic review, whether or not meta-analysis (statistical synthesis) is a component of the review. Data collection includes all methods used to identify published and unpublished data to be included in the review, to determine eligibility of the data for inclusion, and to extract data for analysis. Much of the methodological research related to meta-analysis has, to date, related to statistical methods, not to data collection.[1] It is clear, however, that the validity of the results of statistical analyses depends on the validity of the underlying data.

Unbiased and complete identification of studies is particularly important. Studies relevant for inclusion in a systematic review may not have been published, for reasons related to the findings (publication bias).[2-5] Even when studies are published, they may be difficult to find.

Our objective in the research we describe here was to examine the sensitivity and precision of searching Medline for randomised clinical trials. In this setting, sensitivity is defined as the proportion of the total number of known trials identified by the search and precision is the proportion of publications retrieved by Medline that are actually randomised clinical trials. We performed a two part study, the first specifically searching for randomised clinical trials in vision research (ophthalmology and optometry), the second study combining the results from the vision study with other similar studies to achieve a better estimate of sensitivity and precision of searching across medical disciplines.

# Methods

*(i)a Searching for randomised clinical trials on vision*

In 1991, in collaboration with the Health Sciences Library at the University of Maryland at Baltimore, we developed a two stage search strategy designed to identify randomised clinical trials in vision research. A clinical trial was defined (by C Meinert, 1991) as any planned therapeutic, diagnostic, or preventive study involving humans comparing concurrently one intervention (drug, device, or procedure) to another intervention, placebo, or no intervention, to determine their relative safety and efficacy. Randomised trials were defined as those in which treatment was truly randomised by using a computer generated list or a random numbers table or in which a quasi-randomisation method, such as assignment to treatment by medical record number, was used. Our overall goal was to develop a register of published trials in vision research. The activities described in this article were related to a pilot study for developing the register; the study was designed to devise the best possible strategy for identifying as high a proportion as possible of published randomised clinical trials.

The first search of Medline for reports of randomised clinical trials published in 1988 was relatively broad both in terms of the subject matter covered and the methodological MeSH (medical subject heading) terms (details of strategies used in this study are available from the first author). Citations and abstracts retrieved

19

by the first search were reviewed, and potentially relevant trials were downloaded into Pro-Cite version 1.41 using Biblio-Links.

To determine the "gold standard," all journals that had appeared at least once in the first Medline search results (44 journals) were selected for hand searching for articles reporting randomised clinical trials of research on vision. Thirty nine of the 44 journals were available in local libraries. An additional 27 ophthalmology and optometry journals were selected for hand searching because they included English abstracts and were available in local libraries. Fourteen of these journals were not indexed in Medline. Thus a total of 66 journals were hand searched and reports of randomised clinical trials photocopied for our files. When it was not clear whether an article described a randomised trial, it was given the benefit of the doubt and included in the initial set of articles we used to refine our search strategy.

In the second part of the vision study we performed an analysis of the text words contained in the title and abstract, and the MeSH terms used to index the reports found by the first Medline search and hand searching. This information was used to devise a second Medline search strategy, designed to be more sensitive than the first. The list of references retrieved was reviewed, and new trials were identified and their reports retrieved from the library. These reports together with those identified initially were reviewed by two of us (RS and KD) independently for inclusion in the gold standard.

We further tested the second Medline search strategy by applying it to articles published in 1989. Subsequently, we hand searched for 1989 the four journals publishing the greatest number of randomised clinical trials on vision in our 1988 gold standard.

### (i)b Additional information and analysis

There were two situations in which it was not clear whether an article described a randomised trial. In the first, when articles were published in languages other than those we read, we had the article translated to the degree necessary to determine whether it met our definition of a randomised clinical trial. In the second, when it was not clear from the written report whether a random (or quasi-random) method had been used to allocate patients to an intervention, addresses were obtained and letters requesting this information were written to the first authors of the reports. Second and succeeding authors were written to if no address was available for the first author. If the author stated that the trial used a specific method to randomly assign patients to treatment the report was included in the gold standard. We made no attempt to verify statements in published reports.

We compared the 1988 results of our first and second Medline searches with the gold standard to calculate the sensitivity and precision of the searches. For 1989 reports, we compared the results of the search with the 1989 gold standard compiled by hand searching the four journals. Preliminary results of our search[6][7] have here been updated subsequent to translation of articles and correspondence with authors.

## (ii) Systematic review of studies of searching

*Identification of studies*—We included only articles that reported the results of searches for randomised clinical trials confirmed either in the methods section or by correspondence with the author(s). Our focus on trials is related to our interest in systematic reviews of trials evaluating selected interventions. Several published studies on the sensitivity of Medline searching which were not limited to searching for randomised clinical trials were therefore not included.

We identified studies for our review by using both formal and ad hoc methods. Because of our interest in the problem of Medline searching, one of us (KD) has conducted Medline searches over the years to identify relevant articles. These search strategies have not been standardised; rather, they have depended on the use of text words such as "Medline" and "searching." Bibliographies of these and other related articles have been reviewed for pertinent reports. For this review, CL performed a formal search of Medline and Embase for articles not previously identified. Also, through an international meeting of investigators who conducted original research in this area, convened in November 1992 at the UK Cochrane Centre in Oxford, we learned of new publications not identified using the other methods described.

Letters were written to authors of studies when additional data or clarifications were needed for our analyses. Thus, some information relating to studies in this systematic review may not have been published previously or may differ slightly from that in the published article.

*Gold standard*—The studies included in the review varied somewhat in their approach, but all compared the results of a Medline search to a gold standard of known, published randomised trials. There were three types of gold standard based on known published trials: trial reports published in journals, books, or proceedings, including publications not indexed by Medline; trial reports published in journals indexed in Medline; and trial reports published in selected Medline journals. For example, the searches for randomised clinical trials of intraventricular haemorrhage and neonatal hyperbilirubinaemia[8] used the Oxford Database of Perinatal Trials, which included trial reports from a variety of sources as the gold standard. On the other hand, searches for pain trials[9] focused on seven selected journals covered by Medline; this gold standard was developed by hand searching these journals back to 1966.

In several cases authors of individual studies excluded articles from the numerator (number of studies identified) of the sensitivity and precision calculations because certain criteria for the review were not met. For example, criteria in Dickersin *et al* required articles in English, published between 1966 and 1983.[8] In such cases, articles not meeting the study criteria were also excluded from the denominator (either the gold standard or the number of citations identified by a search). Two studies reported cases where articles should have been included in the Medline database, by virtue of being published in a journal indexed for Medline, but were not.[10 11] In such cases, these articles were allowed to remain in the Medline gold standards, even though they were not in the Medline file.

*Analyses*—Analyses compared the sensitivity and precision of results of the Medline search for the individual studies and combined these findings by adding numerators and denominators to obtain weighted means. When an article described the results of multiple search strategies we used the results from the strategy providing the highest sensitivity, and used estimates of precision derived from that strategy. In two cases, a second group of investigators replicated a search and came up with a strategy that improved the sensitivity of the search (Poynard and Conn[12] and

Bernstein[13]; Silagy[14] and Jadad and McQuay[15]); we reported only the higher sensitivity, where the denominators (gold standards) were identical. Since there was 100% concordance in the gold standards used by Silagy and Jadad and McQuay, and a single sensitivity was extracted for our meta-analysis, we considered these articles to represent a single "study."

We also explored the individual search strategies in an effort to understand differences in retrieval rates. Possible reasons for less than optimal sensitivity were classified into five broad categories: limited use of subject matter MeSH terms; limited use of methodological controlled vocabulary (MeSH, check tags, and publication types); limited use of freetext subject matter terms; limited use of freetext methodological terms; and limited use of truncation.

## Results

### (i) Searching for randomised clinical trials on vision

The gold standard for randomised clinical trials on vision published in 1988, developed by using a combination of hand search and Medline search, comprised a total of 236 reports classified as randomised clinical trials (table 3.1). Forty eight of the reports (20%) were in languages other than English; 222 (94%) were published in Medline journals and 14 (6%) elsewhere.

The first Medline search for articles published in 1988 resulted in 219 references, of which 105 were classified as randomised clinical trials (table 3.2)—a precision of 48%. The sensitivity of the first Medline search was 44% (105/236) in comparison with the gold standard that included all randomised clinical trials published in any journal, and 47% (105/222) for trials reported in Medline journals.

Table 3.1 *"Gold standard" for randomised clinical trials in vision research published in 1988: number (percentage) of reports of randomised clinical trials in Medline and non-Medline journals by language*

| Language | Medline journals | Non-Medline journals | Total |
|----------|------------------|----------------------|-----------|
| English | 183 (82) | 5 (36) | 188 (80) |
| Other | 39 (18) | 9 (64) | 48 (20) |
| Total | 222 (100) | 14 (100) | 236 (100) |

Table 3.2 *Sensitivity and precision of Medline searches for randomised clinical trials of research on vision*

| | No of citations | No of randomised clinical trials found | Precision (%) | Sensitivity (%) | | |
|---|---|---|---|---|---|---|
| | | | | Overall (n = 236) | Medline journals (n = 222) | Selected journals (n = 61) |
| 1988: | | | | | | |
| Search 1 | 219 | 105 | 48 | 44 | 47 | |
| Search 2 | 1520 | 193 | 13 | 82 | 87 | |
| 1989*: | | | | | | |
| Search 2 | 272 | 54 | 20 | | | 88 |

* Four journals searched.

The second Medline search resulted in 1520 references, of which 193 were identified as randomised clinical trials (precision = 13%). Sensitivity of the search using all known randomised clinical trials as the gold standard was 82% and sensitivity using only trials listed in Medline was 87%. The second search identified eight trials missed by both the first Medline search and the hand searches, as well as 24 trials appearing in 17 journals not originally hand searched. A hand search of four of these journals (those that contained more than one citation) resulted in no further additions.

The results of the Medline search for articles published in the four selected journals in 1989, using the second strategy, were similar to those for 1988 in terms of sensitivity. Sixty one reports classified as randomised clinical trials and published in one of the four journals comprised the gold standard. The Medline search retrieved 272 citations for the four journals, of which 54 were confirmed as randomised clinical trials (precision = 20%, sensitivity = 88%).

## (ii) Systematic review

For our review, we identified 12 relevant articles published in journals,[8-10 12-20] data from three studies not yet published at the time of our review,[11 21 22] and data from the first part of our study, reported above (referred to in tables 3.3–3.5 as Dickersin 1994). In each case, investigators performed Medline searches and compared the results of the searches with various gold standards of known trials.

Of the 16 studies identified that examined Medline searching for randomised clinical trials, we obtained information useful for this review from 15. On average, the studies indicated that a Medline search, even when conducted by a trained searcher, yielded only 51% of all known trials (range 17-82%; table 3.3). With a gold standard of only those trials in journals available on Medline, sensitivity was better but still disappointing, at 77%, and for studies that used specially selected Medline journals as a gold standard the weighted average sensitivity was 63% (46-88%).

Some of the studies that investigated the sensitivity of Medline searching also examined strategies that would maximise sensitivity while minimising the number of citations that would have to

Table 3.3 *"Best" sensitivity of Medline searches**

| | | | Proportion (of "gold standard") identified (%) | | |
|---|---|---|---|---|---|
| Year | First author | Topic | Any publication | Any Medline journal | Select Medline journals |
| 1985 | Dickersin | Intraventricular haemorrhage | (19/34) 56 | (19/32) 59 | |
| | | Hyperbilirubinaemia | (28/96) 29 | (28/88) 32 | |
| 1985 | Poynard** | Liver disease | (107/279) 38 | | |
| 1988 | Bernstein** | Liver disease | | (155/195) 79 | |
| 1989 | Ohlsson | Pregnancy | (10/13) 77 | (10/11) 91 | |
| 1990 | Hofmans | Acupuncture | (57/98) 58 | (56/67) 85 | |
| 1991 | Gøtzsche | Rheumatoid arthritis | (128/200) 64 | (128/140) 91 | |
| 1992 | Kleijnen | Homoeopathy | (18/107) 17 | (18/23) 78 | |
| | | Vitamin C | (22/61) 36 | (22/28) 78 | |
| | | Ginkgo | (14/45) 31 | (14/18) 78 | |
| 1994 | Dickersin | Ophthalmology | (193/236) 82 | (193/222) 87 | |
| 1988 | Lacy† | Newborn | (8/17) 47 | (8/17) 47 | |
| 1989 | Kirpalani | Newborn | | | (28/53) 53 |
| 1993 | Jadad | Pain | | | (126/153) 82 |
| 1993 | Jadad/Silagy | Primary care | | | (179/204) 88 |
| 1994 | Dickersin | Ophthalmology | | | (54/61) 88 |
| 1994 | Adams | Mental health | | | (388/746) 52 |
| 1994 | Solomon | Surgery | | | (17/37) 46 |
| (Totals) Weighted means | | | (604/1186) 51 | (651/841) 77 | (792/1254) 63 |
| Range | | | 17-82 | 32-91 | 46-88 |

* Some numbers may vary from publication because clarified by communication with author.
**Same search team and subject
† Unpublished

be reviewed for potential relevance. The results of these studies show that there is wide variation in the precision that can be achieved in searching. For some topics, thousands of citations must be examined to achieve acceptable sensitivity; for others, a relatively small number of citations require review (median precision 32·5% (2-82%); table 3.4).

The differences in the sensitivities achieved with searching may be due to earlier studies having limited their use of subject matter MeSH terms too severely, either in the area of subheadings[12] of other related terms[18 19] (table 3.5). Other common deficiencies are limited use of free text terms and limited use of truncated text terms.

Table 3.4 *Precision of Medline searches (proportion of trials retrieved that are relevant)*

| Year | First author | Topic | No of relevant trials | No retrieved | % of relevant trials |
|------|------|------|------|------|------|
| | | *Any Medline journal* | | | |
| 1985 | Dickersin | Intraventricular haemorrhage | 19 | 36 | 53 |
| | | Hyperbilirubi-naemia | 28 | 39 | 72 |
| 1988 | Bernstein | Liver disease | 155 | 9 643 | 2 |
| 1989 | Ohlsson | Pregnancy | 10 | 125 | 8 |
| 1991 | Gøtzsche | Rheumatoid ar-thritis | 128 | 738 | 17 |
| 1992 | Kleijnen | Homoeopathy | 18 | 52 | 35 |
| | | Vitamin C | 22 | 81 | 27 |
| | | Ginkgo | 14 | 46 | 30 |
| 1994 | Dickersin | Ophthalmology | 193 | 1 520 | 13 |
| 1988 | Lacy† | Newborn | 8 | 21 | 38 |
| Total (weighted mean; median) | | | 595 | 12 301 | (5; 29) |
| | | *Select Medline journals* | | | |
| 1989 | Kirpalani | Newborn | 28 | 34 | 82 |
| 1993 | Jadad | Pain | 126 | 245 | 51 |
| 1994 | Dickersin | Ophthalmology | 54 | 272 | 20 |
| 1994 | Adams | Mental health | 388 | 662 | 59 |
| Total (weighted mean: median) | | | 596 | 1 213 | (49; 55) |
| Grand total (weighted mean; median) Range | | | 1 191 | 13 514 | (9; 33) (2%-82%) |

† Unpublished

Table 3.5 *Possible reasons for non-optimal sensitivity of "best" Medline searches*

| Year | First author | Limited use of MeSH terms | | Limited use of free text terms | | Limited use of truncated text terms |
|---|---|---|---|---|---|---|
| | | Subject matter | Methods | Subject matter | Methods | |
| 1985 | Dickersin | | | ✓ | | |
| 1985 | Poynard | ✓ | ✓ | ✓ | ✓ | ✓ |
| 1988 | Bernstein | | | ✓ | | ✓ |
| 1989 | Kirpalani | ✓ | | ✓ | | ✓ |
| 1989 | Ohlsson | ✓ | | ✓ | | ✓ |
| 1990 | Hofmans | ✓ | ✓ | ✓ | ✓ | ✓ |
| 1991 | Gøtzsche | | | ✓ | | ✓ |
| 1992 | Kleijnen | | | ✓ | ✓ | ✓ |
| 1993 | Jadad | | | | | ✓ |
| 1993 | Jadad/Silagy | | | | | |
| 1994 | Dickersin | | | | | ✓ |
| 1994 | Adams | * | | * | | |
| Unpublished | Lacy | | No data | ✓ | No data | ✓ |
| 1994 | Solomon | | | ✓ | | ✓ |

*Adams *et al* did not use any "subject" terms in their search strategy. Instead they used journal title to restrict their retrieval.

## Discussion

The sensitivity of Medline is 51% when the gold standard is all known randomised clinical trials published in journals indexed in Medline and in those not indexed in Medline. Thus, if comprehensive systematic reviews of randomised clinical trials depend solely on Medline searches they will omit about half of the available studies. It is not even possible to identify all the published trials in journals indexed in Medline by using Medline (weighted mean = 77%).

There are about 22 000 active medical serial titles,[23] of which about 16 000 can be classified as journals; only about 3700 of these are in Medline. Not all 16 000 journals are likely to publish the reports of randomised trials, but many include the results of randomised clinical trials presented at meetings, only half of which ever reach full publication.[24] It might be argued that the quality of reports in non-Medline journals is lower than that of reports in Medline journals and thus that missing randomised clinical trials reported in non-Medline journals in a systematic review might be relatively unimportant—but there is no evidence that this is so.

### Inadequate indexing

Sensitivity was much better, about 77%, on comparison of the results of Medline searching only with a gold standard of known randomised clinical trials that are included in the Medline file. This proportion could and should be 100%; the problem results mainly from inadequate indexing, for which there are several reasons. Firstly, until fairly recently there has been an emphasis on developing MeSH terms for subject matter rather than methodology. For example, there was no suitable descriptor term to describe randomisation as a methodology until RANDOM ALLOCATION was introduced in 1978. RANDOMIZED CONTROLLED TRIALS was introduced in 1990 as a descriptor term and RANDOMIZED CONTROLLED TRIAL was introduced in 1991 as a publication type. Secondly, even when suitable descriptor terms were available, they have not been and continue not to be applied consistently by indexers acting for the National Library of Medicine (P L Schuyler et al, second international congress on peer review, 1993; C Lefebvre et al, conference on "An evidence-based health care system: the case for clinical trial registries" at National Institutes of Health, 1993). Thirdly, authors may not have described their research methods clearly enough to allow accurate indexing of methodology. For example, 11% (25/236) of the trials comprising the broadest gold standard in vision research could not be verified as randomised clinical trials by readers and required confirmation by a letter to the author. For an additional 37 articles, the authors did not respond to inquiries or could not be reached. These articles may have been randomised clinical trials but could not be included in the gold standard because their status remains unclear.

### Factors affecting sensitivity and precision

The calculation of sensitivity requires comparing the results of a Medline search with known randomised clinical trials. Two major factors will influence this calculation. The first is the comprehensiveness of the gold standard. It is likely that the more comprehensive the gold standard, the less sensitive the Medline search, particularly if the gold standard includes many randomised clinical trials in journals not indexed in Medline. Thus, differences across studies in sensitivity may be related to the completeness of the gold standard or of the field itself. We examined the available data by using three possible gold standards, so the sensitivities presented address different questions. The sensitivity of searches using trial reports from any publication as a denominator expresses, at least theoretically, the probability of identifying all published randomised clinical trials in a field, although few gold standards are likely to be complete. The sensitivity of searches using reports from any Medline journal as a denominator expresses the probability of identifying randomised clinical trials known to be available on Medline. Assuming the investigators have done a thorough job, this gold standard is more likely to be "complete" because the universe of trials indexed in Medline is well defined. The gold standard using selected Medline journals can be easily checked for reliability and validity because it uses a specific subset of journals published within a defined time period. If the journals included in this gold standard were representative of all journals over all time periods it would provide an estimate of the overall sensitivity of Medline searching. It is not likely to be representative, however, and thus its chief value is that the denominator of the sensitivity calculation (the gold standard) is likely to be accurate.

The second factor influencing the calculation of sensitivity and precision estimates is the quality of the Medline search. Because Medline is a highly structured database with complex indexing rules, a certain level of skill and experience is necessary to achieve good (sensitive and precise) results. Untrained Medline searchers are unlikely to find a high proportion of all the relevant references. Any effort to increase the number of relevant references retrieved is likely to be at the expense of precision, so that an unacceptably high proportion of irrelevant references may need to be reviewed.

Our systematic review indicates that Medline searching for randomised clinical trials achieves a median precision of about 33%. Sensitivity was highest when precision was at or below 35%, and decreased as precision increased (figure 3.1). The point at which to balance precision and sensitivity must be decided by the individuals performing the systematic reviews. For example, some studies included in our review knowingly omitted terms that would have increased sensitivity (COMPARATIVE STUDY, for example) because precision would have been severely compromised. Sensitivity may also vary within subject matter categories

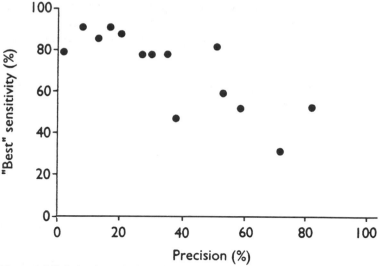

Figure 3.1 Relation between "best" sensitivity (gold standard obtained for either any journal indexed by Medline or selected Medline journals) and precision for Medline searching of 14 topics

and journals searched, although this has not been examined systematically.

*Languages*

From the study of searching for vision trials, we learned that 18% of the relevant Medline articles and 20% overall were not in English. Most (29/37) of the articles that remained unclassified were not reported in English. The proportion of randomised clinical trials overall that are written in languages other than English is no doubt higher than our experience from Medline suggests. Had we searched Embase (the Reed-Elsevier Excerpta Medica database), which includes many European language journals not indexed for Medline, we would undoubtedly have identified additional trials in other languages (see chapter 2). These findings imply that excluding from a meta-analysis studies published in languages other than English or limiting a search to Medline will result in more than a trivial number of studies being omitted. A comprehensive search of several databases and non-English publications may lead to considerable translation expenses, depending on the project undertaken. Whether an article reports a randomised clinical trial may not be apparent even after an article has been translated. We recommend not translating the entire article until someone who is able to read the language ascertains that it is or may possibly be a randomised clinical trial.

### Improving retrieval through Medline

Retrieval of randomised clinical trials through Medline can be improved in three ways:

improve terminology used in reports so that it is clear that they describe the results of a randomised clinical trial;

improve indexing so that all randomised clinical trials are indexed with the appropriate publication type term RANDOMIZED CONTROLLED TRIAL; and

improve strategies used to search for randomised clinical trials. Use of truncation and both subject matter and methods textwords are particularly important.

The first strategy relies on editors taking the lead. Until editors require adequate descriptions of study methodology in the title or abstract, as well as the methods section, of every article published we cannot expect adequate indexing. Indexers can apply a study design term only if authors explicitly describe the design. For example, a tag of RANDOMIZED CONTROLLED TRIAL cannot be applied if authors never state that the study was randomised. Authors and editors must consider the indexing when they are writing, taking special care that the title and abstract are informative and precise; use of structured abstracts should facilitate this.

Improved indexing relies on training and quality measures taken by the National Library of Medicine and also on the availability of indexing terms. Recent changes in Medline indexing should result in more sensitive searches in the future.

Searchers can improve retrieval of randomised clinical trials from Medline in several ways. In our vision study we used a two stage search strategy. We searched one year first, identified the journals that published randomised clinical trials, hand searched those journals for a single year, identified additional MeSH and freetext terms that would have proved useful in identifying articles, and performed a second Medline search incorporating these new terms. Hand searching journals (in our study, 66 journals for 1988) to create a gold standard might seem daunting, but it does provide information on the indexing of the randomised clinical trials that were not picked up by the first search.

Modifications of this approach are possible. For example, one could combine the results of a first Medline search with trials identified by other means (for example, review of lists of references incorporated in reports of trials identified by the first search). Jadad and McQuay suggest that combining a Medline search with a selective hand search just of published conference abstracts (such as are found in journal supplements) and letters is a reasonable approach when funds for hand searching are limited.[9] More research is needed as to whether performing a two stage search, such as described here, or a single Medline search plus hand search will achieve a similar sensitivity.

Advances have been made in developing new searching strategies, primarily through comparison of existing strategies and their results. Our review of the strategies used for 12 of the 15 studies included in our meta-analysis found that limited use of textword searching was the most consistent defect. (Our evaluation is potentially biased, however, because we are also authors or advisers on search strategies designed for several of the articles included in the systematic review.)

## Unpublished trials

Improving Medline searching does not address the issue of how best to identify the 25-50% of trials started but never published,[25] or the problem of identifying reports published in non-Medline journals. Linking international databases (Medline and Embase, for example) may help. In addition, access to "grey" literature (literature not formally published, such as research reports, policy documents, dissertations, and conference abstracts) remains difficult (see chapter 2). The advent of specific grey literature databases such as SIGLE, produced by the European Association for Grey Literature (a group of national information and documentation centres devoted to providing access to such literature) has improved the situation, but much research remains inaccessible. The literature is not insignficant, and trials reported there may not see full publication elsewhere: on average, only 50% of abstracts reporting the results of randomised clinical trials reach full publication.[24]

Although some authors advocate not making the effort to identify unpublished trials because the data have not undergone peer review,[26] excluding data from unpublished trials will lead to a loss in precision of the estimate of an effect size. In addition, failure to publish is associated with "negative" results (results that are not statistically significant); this association results in a publication bias.[25] Publication bias has serious implications for unbiased data collection for a systematic review. Publication bias extends beyond the failure to publish a report: Stewart and Parmar found that data are selectively omitted from published articles, and they recommend that all systematic reviews be based on data on individual patients rather than published reports (see also chapter 4).[27] The conditions required for this approach, however, are not available to most reviewers.

Those planning to undertake meta-analyses should not under-estimate the difficulty or expense of performing a well conducted systematic review. There is no question that the choice of methods used for data collection is the key to the validity of such a review. Right now, the only alternatives to electronic searching are development of trials registers and use of hand search. Both are costly. But if health care is to be based on all available evidence rather than selected evidence, these costs must be borne or the reviews may be misleading.

*Registers of randomised clinical trials*

Systems for registration of trials should be available to facilitate unbiased data collection for systematic reviews. We are currently participating in the Cochrane Collaboration[28] and are in the process of developing such a register in collaboration with the National Library of Medicine. Cooperation from investigators and journal editors, as well as support from funding agencies, will be needed to make this effort a success.

The first step is to identify all published randomised clinical trials through electronic and hand searching of the literature. We have devised a generalised search strategy (Appendix), based on the results of this review, that will be used to develop the core of the register. The strategy is in three stages: stage one (sets 1-8) includes terms with high precision, stage two (sets 9-24) includes terms with moderate precision, and stage three (sets 25-34) includes terms with low precision but which provide optimal sensitivity. Each stage is limited to exclude reports solely of animal studies, but retains reports indexed as human and animal, and neither human nor animal.

Journal editors are being asked to arrange for hand searches of their own journals to ensure that all randomised clinical trials published in them will be included in the register and thus will have the best opportunity for inclusion in systematic reviews. The Baltimore Cochrane Centre is coordinating the activities involved in identifying reports of randomised controlled trials and ensuring that these reports are forwarded to the National Library of Medicine for retagging with an appropriate "publication type" term. In addition to the existing publication type term RANDOMIZED CONTROLLED TRIAL, which was introduced in 1991, the National Library of Medicine has agreed to introduce a new publication type term, CONTROLLED CLINICAL TRIAL, from January 1995. This will be used to tag all reports in Medline that meet the Cochrane Collaboration's criteria for defining a controlled trial but do not meet the library's criteria for indexing under the more specific term RANDOMIZED CONTROLLED TRIAL. Both terms will be applied retrospectively to reports identified by the electronic and handsearching activities described above. Tagging with the new term should become less important as editors insist on explicit descriptions of study methodology which will enable accurate tagging with RANDOMIZED CONTROLLED TRIAL.

The second step of development is prospective registration of all randomised clinical trials. Many trial registers in specific subject areas already exist,[29][30] and the International Collaborative Group on Clinical Trials Registries has been working towards such a goal for several years.[31]

The National Institutes of Health sponsored an international conference in December 1993 entitled "An evidence-based health care system: the case for clinical trial registries," focusing on all aspects of trial registration and bringing together many of the leaders in this field. There is considerable optimism that the scientific, medical, and information communities are moving towards a situation in which unbiased data collection for systematic reviews will become more possible. The implications for evidence based health care are great.

1 Dickersin K, Berlin J. Meta-analysis: state-of-the-science. *Epidemiol Rev* 1992; 14: 154–76.
2 Dickersin K, Chan S, Chalmers TC, Sacks HS, Smith H Jr. Publication bias and clinical trials. *Controlled Clin Trials* 1987; 8: 343–53.
3 Easterbrook PJ, Berlin JA, Gopalan R, Matthews DW. Publication bias in clinical research. *Lancet* 1991; 337: 867–72.
4 Dickersin K, Min YI, Meinert CL. Factors influencing publication of research results: follow-up of applications submitted to two institutional review boards. *JAMA* 1992; 263: 374–8.

# IDENTIFYING RELEVANT STUDIES FOR SYSTEMATIC REVIEWS

5  Dickersin K, Min YI. NIH clinical trials and publication bias. *Online J Curr Clin Trials* [serial online] 1993 Apr 28; Doc No 50: 4967 words; 53 paragraphs.

6  Scherer R, Dickersin K, Kaplan E, Min TI. Initiation of a registry of randomized clinical trials in vision research. *Invest Ophthalmol Vis Sci* 1992; 33: 1323.

7  Scherer R, Dickersin K, Kaplan E. The accessible biomedical literature represents a fraction of all studies in a field. In: Weeks RA, Kinser DL (eds). *Editing the refereed scientific journal*. New York: IEEE Press, 1994; 24: 120–5.

8  Dickersin K, Hewitt P, Mutch L, Chalmers I, Chalmers TC. Comparison of Medline searching with a perinatal trials database. *Controlled Clin Trials* 1985; 6: 306–17.

9  Jadad AR, McQuay HJ. A high-yield strategy to identify randomized controlled trials for systematic reviews. *Online J Curr Clin Trials* [serial online] 1993; Doc No 33: 3973 words; 39 paragraphs.

10  Gøtzsche PC, Lange B. Comparison of search strategies for recalling double-blind trials from Medline. *Dan Med Bull* 1991; 38: 476–8.

11  Adams CE, Power A, Frederick K, Lefebvre C. An investigation of the adequacy of Medline searches for randomized controlled trials (RCTs) of the effects of mental health care. *Psychol Med* 1994; 24: 741–8.

12  Poynard T, Conn HO. The retrieval of randomized clinical trials in liver disease from the medical literature. A comparison of MEDLARS and manual methods. *Controlled Clin Trials* 1985; 6: 271–9.

13  Bernstein F. The retrieval of randomized clinical trials in liver diseases from the medical literature: manual versus Medlars searches. *Controlled Clin Trials* 1988; 9: 23–31.

14  Silagy C. Developing a register of randomised controlled trials in primary care. *BMJ* 1993; 306: 897–900.

15  Jadad AR, McQuay IIJ. Be systematic in your searching. *BMJ* 1993; 307: 66.

16  Ohlsson A, Treatments of preterm premature rupture of the membranes: a meta-analysis. *Am J Obstet Gynecol* 1989; 160: 890–906.

17  Daya S. Efficacy of progesterone support for pregnancy in women with recurrent miscarriage. A meta-analysis of controlled trials. *Br J Obstet Gynaecol* 1989; 96: 275–80.

18  Hofmans EA. The results of a Medline search. The accessibility of research on the effectiveness of acupuncture.II. *Huisarts Wet* 1990; 33: 103–6.

19  Kirpalani H, Schmidt B, McKibbon KA, Haynes RB, Sinclair JC. Searching Medline for randomized clinical trials involving care of the newborn. *Pediatrics* 1989; 83: 543–6.

20  Kleijnen J, Knipschild P. The comprehensiveness of Medline and Embase computer searches. Searches for controlled trials of homeopathy, ascorbic acid for common cold and ginkgo biloba for cerebral insufficiency and intermittent claudication. *Pharm Weekbl Scientific Edition* 1992; 14: 316–20.

21  Lacy JB, Ohlsson A. The administration of intravenous immunoglobulins for prophylaxis or treatment of infection in preterm infants: meta-analyses. (Unpublished.)

22  Solomon MJ, Laxamana A, Devore L, McLeod RS. Randomized controlled trials in surgery. *Surgery* 1994; 115: 707–12.

23  United States Department of Health and Human Services, Public Health Service, National Institutes of Health. *Fact sheet, technical services division*. Bethesda, MA: National Library of Medicine, 1993: March.

24  Scherer R, Dickersin K, Langenberg P. Full publication of results initially presented as abstracts: a meta-analysis. *JAMA* 1994; 272: 158–62.

25  Dickersin K, Min YI. Publication bias: the problem that won't go away. *Ann NY Acad Sci* 1993; 703: 135–48.

26  Chalmers TC, Berrier J, Sacks HS, Levin H, Reitman D, Nagalingam P. Meta-analysis of clinical trials as a scientific discipline. II. Replicate variability and comparison of studies that agree and disagree. *Stat Med* 1987; 6: 733–44.

27  Stewart L, Parmar M. Meta-analysis of the literature or of individual patient data: is there a difference? *Lancet* 1993; 341: 418–22.

28  Chalmers I, Dickersin K, Chalmers TC. Getting to grips with Archie Cochrane's agenda. *BMJ* 1992; 305: 786–8.

29  Easterbrook PJ. Directory of registries of clinical trials. *Stat Med* 1992; 11: 345–423.

30  Dickersin K. Why register trials?—revisited. *Controlled Clin Trials* 1992; 13: 170–7.

31  Ad Hoc Working Party of the International Collaborative Group on Clinical Trials Registries. Position paper and consensus recommendations on clinical trial registries. *Clin Trials Meta-analysis* 1993; 28: 255–66.

# Appendix

*Optimally sensitive Medline search strategy for identifying randomised clinical trials*

| Set No | Term searched or sets combined |
|--------|--------------------------------|
| 1 | RANDOMIZED-CONTROLLED-TRIAL in PT |
| 2 | RANDOMIZED-CONTROLLED-TRIALS |
| 3 | RANDOM-ALLOCATION |
| 4 | DOUBLE-BLIND-METHOD |
| 5 | SINGLE-BLIND-METHOD |
| 6 | 1 or 2 or 3 or 4 or 5 |
| 7 | TG=ANIMAL not (TG=HUMAN and TG=ANIMAL) |
| 8 | 6 not 7 |
| | |
| 9 | CLINICAL-TRIAL in PT |
| 10 | explode CLINICAL-TRIALS |
| 11 | (clin* near trial*) in TI |
| 12 | (clin* near trial*) in AB |
| 13 | (singl* or doubl* or trebl* or tripl*) near (blind* or mask*) |
| 14 | (13 in TI) or (13 in AB) |
| 15 | PLACEBOS |
| 16 | placebo* in TI |
| 17 | placebo* in AB |
| 18 | random in TI |
| 19 | random in AB |
| 20 | RESEARCH-DESIGN |
| 21 | 9 or 10 or 11 or 12 or 14 or 15 or 16 or 17 or 18 or 19 or 20 |
| 22 | TG=ANIMAL not (TG=HUMAN and TG=ANIMAL) |
| 23 | 21 not 22 |
| 24 | 23 not 8 |
| | |
| 25 | TG=COMPARATIVE-STUDY |
| 26 | explode EVALUATION-STUDIES |
| 27 | FOLLOW-UP-STUDIES |
| 28 | PROSPECTIVE-STUDIES |
| 29 | control* or prospectiv* or volunteer* |
| 30 | (29 in TI) or (29 in AB) |
| 31 | 25 or 26 or 27 or 28 or 30 |
| 32 | TG=ANIMAL not (TG=HUMAN and TG=ANIMAL) |
| 33 | 31 not 32 |
| 34 | 33 not (8 or 24) |

Format shown is for SilverPlatter version 3.10. Upper case denotes controlled vocabulary; lower case denotes freetext terms. Those wishing to run this search strategy are recommended to seek the advice of a trained medical librarian.

# 4 Obtaining data from randomised controlled trials: how much do we need for reliable and informative meta-analyses?

MICHAEL J CLARKE, LESLEY A STEWART

## Summary

Many randomised controlled trials compare treatments that will produce only moderate differences in outcome, but these differences can be clinically important. However, they are difficult to assess reliably and require a large amount of randomised evidence. This can be achieved through large prospective randomised trials which will accrue future patients, the meta-analysis of results from randomised trials involving patients from the past, or—ideally—both. The techniques require that all possible biases are minimised, and in meta-analyses this can best be achieved by ensuring that all of the randomised evidence—both trials and participants of those trials—is included. The meta-analysis of individual patient data has been described as the yardstick for this approach. It will remove many of the problems associated with relying solely on published data

37

and some of the problems arising from a reliance on aggregate data, and will also add to the analyses that can be performed. Such projects, however, require considerable time and effort.

The differences in outcome between many of the treatments compared in randomised trials are moderate but potentially very important to patients and their medical carers. Individually, however, most trials have been too small to assess such differences reliably. There are two main ways to overcome this: through large prospective randomised trials which will accrue future patients, and through meta-analyses of completed trials. Whether a single randomised trial or a meta-analysis is to be undertaken, all possible biases should be minimised, and perhaps the most important step in this is to ensure that as much as possible of the randomised evidence is included in the analyses.[1]

This paper sets out the reasons for and the means of doing this. It emphasises meta-analysis using individual patient data, which has been described[2] as a yardstick against which other forms of systematic review could be measured, but many of the points raised are also relevant to meta-analyses using aggregate data. The individual patient data approach requires that data on every patient entered to all relevant randomised trials are collected centrally, allowing careful data checking and standard analyses to be performed, and an overall result, based on the totality of the available evidence, to be calculated. These projects can provide reliable evidence in areas of uncertainty, as in the Early Breast Cancer Trialists' Collaborative Group's meta-analyses of randomised trials of tamoxifen and chemotherapy[3][4] and the Non-Small Cell Lung Cancer Collaborators Group's meta-analyses of chemotherapy.[5]

Several other such projects have been undertaken successfully and the little quantitative and empirical evidence published to date has shown their advantages over reviews based on published or aggregate data alone[6][7]. These advantages arise because of the increased accuracy and updating of the material available for review and the additional analyses that are possible with individual patient data but cannot be done with aggregate data alone. Some of the advantages of collecting individual patient data are described below, along with suggestions on how such data may be collected. This work is based on the practical experience of two of the groups who have acted as secretariats for some of the largest meta-analyses based on individual patient data conducted to date. (To expand this experience, a workshop was organised recently by the Cochrane Collaboration to bring together representatives of other groups undertaking such projects. A full report of the findings of the workshop, including areas such as protocol use and development, methods of checking data, and resource requirements is available from the authors.)

## Minimising biases and random errors

### Complete identification of published and unpublished trials

The most important step in the conduct of any systematic review of randomised controlled trials is to identify and include all (or nearly all) of the relevant trials. This is needed whether the review is to be based on aggregate or individual patient data; the process of trial identification is described in the previous chapter.[8] Meta-analyses based on individual patient data always require direct contact with trialists (as do some reviews based on aggregate data), so these provide an additional means of identifying trials—enlisting the help and knowledge of those trialists. For example, neither of two important reviews of randomised trials comparing melphalan and prednisone with combination chemotherapy in the treatment of multiple myeloma[9][10] found the unpublished Italian M-80 randomised trial of these drugs versus vincristine plus melphalan, cyclophosphamide, and prednisone. This study was also unknown to the secretariat of an ongoing overview of such trials until the Italian group was contacted for patient data from its other trials. Similarly, direct contact with trialists identified two unpublished trials previously unknown to the secretariat of a meta-analysis of advanced ovarian cancer[11]; these had not been identified by a meta-analyses based on the published literature.

### Obtaining information on all randomised participants and excluding information on those who were not randomised.

All randomised patients should be included in the analysis in accordance with the treatment allocated at randomisation (an "intention to treat" analysis). In this way, the policy of using one treatment will be appropriately compared with the policy of using another.[12] Unfortunately, many randomised trials do not follow this principle when publishing their results, and patients are excluded for a variety of reasons. Sometimes these reasons will seem unconnected with the assigned treatment—for example, when the delayed result of a prerandomisation diagnostic test reveals that the patient was ineligible for the study. More seriously, the reasons can be related to treatment—for example, the patient may have been unable to tolerate the allocated treatment or failed to follow the treatment schedule for some other reason.

Many published papers will state that some patients have been judged ineligible and omitted from the analyses, and the people reading the paper will be aware of the size of the problems this might cause. A more difficult problem arises if a publication contains no mention of randomised but ineligible patients, usually because the trialist considers that these patients are no longer part of the trial. Such a situation was noted recently by Hoover *et al* for their randomised trial of active-specific immunotherapy in colorectal cancer. The second publication[13] of this study's results noted that an oversight in an earlier publication[14] led to the failure to state that some patients were randomised but excluded from the analyses.

Occasionally, some non-randomised patients are included in a trial's published analyses—then it is important that these patients are excluded from the meta-analysis. This can happen if a randomised trial was preceded by a non-randomised run in phase, or if patients continue to be entered to one of the study's treatments after the randomisation has been closed. It can also happen if the randomisation is temporarily stopped during the trial. Figure 4.1 shows this for an unpublished trial of radiotherapy versus chemotherapy in multiple myeloma. The radiotherapy equipment was not available for six months during the trial, but patients continued to enter the chemotherapy arm. The appropriate analysis of the trial would exlude this group of patients, but it was only when the data were supplied for the overview that the problem was brought back to the attention of the trialist.

*Obtaining complete and unbiased information on all subgroups and outcomes studied*

A trial that collects information on a variety of patient

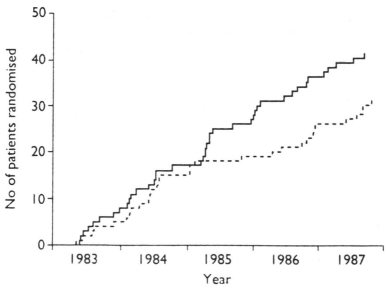

Figure 4.1 Entry of patients to randomised trial showing accrual of patients to chemotherapy (and radiotherapy) treatment groups. Individual patient data include patients entered to the chemotherapy group during April to September 1985, when radiotherapy was not available, these patients should not be included in the meta-analysis. (Figure included with permission of trialist)

characteristics can have as many subgroup analyses as there are types of patient in the data. Whether or not these analyses provide useful information will not be debated here. Constraints on space and other influences make it most likely that the analyses relating to the subgroups with the most striking results will be published. Thus, any subgroup analyses in a systematic review that uses only those subgroups available in published reports will be subject to both the effect of publication bias in the trials available for inclusion and an additional bias in the subgroups available for analysis.

Similarly, if a trial measures several outcome measures there will be a tendency for those showing the most striking results to be published. This could occur if a series of alternative measures is used for the same outcome, such as rating scales in psychiatric illness, or if the outcome measure can vary depending on the convention used to define it, such as event free survival in leukaemia.

The collection of unpublished material helps with this in two

41

main ways. If the patient characteristics are obtained for all trials, subgroup analyses based on the total evidence can be performed. Moreover, these analyses will contain a larger number of events and have greater statistical power than any single trial.

With regard to outcome measures, it may be possible to specify a uniform definition for a particular outcome and analyse this across all trials. It is worth remembering that whether or not a subgroup or outcome can be analysed will depend on its initial collection by the trialist (a decision that could not have been biased by the trial's own results) and on the willingness of the trialist to supply data on that variable—a problem that can happen with any of the data or trials in the meta-analysis.

### Obtaining complete follow up data

Whenever the results of a trial are published, those results become "frozen in time" and will usually remain so unless the trial is updated and published again, which happens rarely. The supply of information for a meta-analysis is another way in which the trial's results can be updated, both by providing additional follow up and by completing data that were missing at the time of publication. The effect of the additional material on the results of a meta-analysis will vary. For example, an overview of the comparison of single non-platinum drugs with platinum-based combination chemotherapy in advanced ovarian cancer found that increasing the period of follow up reduced the estimate of the overall treatment benefit.[6] In contrast, the breast cancer overview found an additional benefit for patients allocated to adjuvant chemotherapy, rather than control, when the follow up was extended and standardised to the period 5-10 years after treatment.[4] This result was so surprising to the statistical secretariat at the time of the preliminary analyses that a questionnaire was sent to all of the collaborating trialists. Seventy eight replied and their predictions for the additional effect of prolonged multiagent chemotherapy in premenopausal women during years 5-10 after surgery ranged from an increase in the odds of death of 20% to a decrease of 25%. None were as extreme as the overview result—an additional decrease of 33%.

### How to obtain data that are as complete as possible

Whether the information on the participants in the relevant randomised trials should be collected as aggregate data or individual patient data will be discussed briefly below. In either case, it must be collected from as many eligible trials as possible. It is especially important to ensure that any trials that do not contribute data are not so numerous or unrepresentative as to introduce important bias into the result of the systematic review. Thus the data collection process may present the reviewer with several difficulties. Some trialists may be reluctant to supply their data, and there will often be practical difficulties in preparing data. It is important therefore to emphasise that any data supplied will be treated confidentially and will not be used for any additional purpose without the permission of the responsible trialist. In addition, any publications arising from the meta-analysis should be in the name of all the collaborators, and each trialist should have an opportunity to comment on the manuscript before publication. The trialists will also be the first people, other than the statistical secretariat, to see and discuss the overview results if these are presented first to a closed meeting of the collaborative group of all participating trialists.

If there are trialists who initially were unable to prepare and supply their data, some of these points may help persuade them to do so. In addition, the process of data collection should be as simple and flexible as possible so as to help and encourage trialists to participate. In some instances, even if the initial request was for aggregate data it may be easier and preferable for the trialist to supply individual patient data so that the necessary tables can be prepared centrally. This might be the case if, for example, only paper records exist for each patient in the trial or if the trialist does not have the necessary resources to prepare the tables.

Patience also helps because data that are regarded as completely lost may sometimes reappear. For example, the third cycle of the early breast cancer overview will include a trial whose records were feared lost in a flood at the time of the second cycle, but which were recently found when an office was cleared.

# Benefits of using individual patient data rather than aggregate data

The reasons for obtaining information on all randomised patients in all relevant trials have been described above, and these goals can often be achieved by collecting aggregate information from the responsible trialists. Collecting individual patient data may allow some of them to be achieved more easily or reliably and will also provide important additional benefits.

### Calculation of times to events

Perhaps the most substantial benefit is that it is not possible to calculate and analyse the times to specific events reliably without individual patient data. Such analyses might reveal prolongation of event free periods or differences in median survival for the treatments being compared. Figure 4.2 shows hypothetical

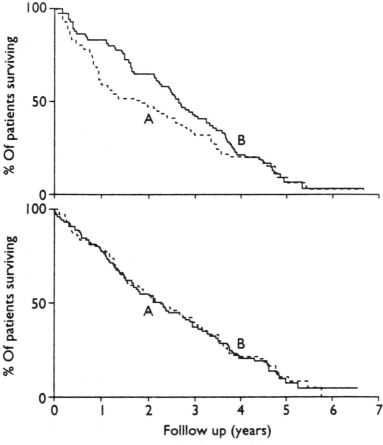

Figure 4.2 Simulated survival curves with approximately the same survival in both groups at 4 years (B) but not at 2 years (A)

examples of how the divergence of the survival curves, which might be of great relevance to patients and clinicians, would be missed if aggregate data were collected for any time beyond point B. Data collected only for time A would produce an over-optimistic conclusion on the treatment benefit in the upper example. In addition, the time to event analyses contribute greater statistical power than is possible with the limited number of time points that would be available with aggregate data.

### Checking and correcting data

Although our experience after looking at data from hundreds of trials is that deliberate fraud in randomised controlled trials is rare, the requirement for individual patient data can help to serve as a check on the use of fabricated data, either from a complete trial or part of a trial. Much more commonly, the central review of patient data will highlight problems with a randomised trial that occurred through error rather than fraud. These mostly arise during the process of randomisation itself or in the follow up of patients in the treatment groups.

For example, the individual patient data might reveal the exclusion of randomised participants or the inclusion of some who were not randomised. This would come to light if the data provided contain a different number of patients from that reported for a trial or if there were sequence gaps due to the absence of some patients. In either case the data on the missing patients could then be requested from the trialist, or the inclusion of additional non-randomised patients could be queried. The patient data will also reveal if patients who were inappropriately classified as ineligible have as much follow up information as eligible patients. If not, the trialist can be asked for further information. Once all of the data are available, the appropriate intention to treat analysis can be performed.

### Supply of additional patient data

If individual patient data are collected it is relatively easy for a trialist to supply additional follow up information or previously missing data on selected patients and for this to be incorporated in the meta-analysis, but if aggregate data were collected the trialist would have to produce a new set of tables. In meta-analyses where death is a major end point, the individual patient data may also allow the central secretariat to continue the follow up through national death registers.

*More flexible and powerful analysis of subgroups and outcome measures.*

If subgroup analyses are to be performed and different outcome measures are to be used, the complexity of the summary tables might become such that they resembled individual patient data. For example, having seven important categories of patient, two important outcome measures and a randomisation into two groups would result in a table with 28 separate values. This is the minimum that would have been required for one table of results in the report of the overview of systemic treatment versus control in breast cancer, which contained the recurrence free and overall survival results among women above and below 50 years of age, with and without nodal involvement, who had positive, negative, or unknown oestrogen receptor status.[4] In addition, because the outcome data will amost certainly be needed for more than one point in time, the aggregate data must be produced for each of these points.

*Other advantages of the collaborative effort*

The involvement of a group of trialists in a meta-analysis can provide wide experience and helpful input when the results are being prepared for publication. The effort involved in collecting and analysing the data can justify holding a collaborators' meeting at which this experience can be expressed and assimilated in a much more interactive way than is possible with the circulation of a draft manuscript. It also allows an additional check that each trialist's data have been properly included in the meta-analysis.

## Conclusion

The most important first step in any systematic review is ensuring that all, or nearly all, relevant trials are identified. After that, the data for analyses can be gathered in a variety of ways. Collecting individual patient data centrally is perhaps the most resource intensive and time consuming of these. This will, however, overcome many of the problems associated with relying solely on published data and some of the problems associated with relying on aggregate data and will add to the analyses that can be performed. It might therefore provide the gold standard to which systematic reviews should strive.[15]

Which steps in the process are the most important for improving reliability requires further testing and evidence, especially if some of these steps lengthen the time needed to conduct the meta-analysis but do not greatly improve its reliability. To this end, some topics for consideration would be the use of trials from which individual patient data are not available but published data are and of trials in which the individual patient data reveal problems (such as the inappropriate exclusion of some patients and the subsequent destruction of their relevant records) that cannot be rectified.

Just as different forms of health care need to be reliably assessed, so the techniques for reviewing evidence from randomised controlled trials should be empirically investigated.

1 Peto R, Collins R, Gray R. Large scale randomized evidence: large, simple trials and overviews of trials. *Ann N Y Acad Sci* 1993; 703: 314–40.
2 Chalmers I. The Cochrane Collaboration: preparing, maintaining, and disseminating systematic reviews of the effects of health care. *Ann N Y Acad Sci* 1993; 703: 156–65
3 Review of mortality results in randomised trials in early breast cancer. *Lancet* 1984; ii: 1205.
4 Early Breast Cancer Trialists' Collaborative Group. Systemic treatment of early breast cancer by hormonal, cytotoxic or immune therapy: 133 randomised trials involving 31,000 recurrences and 24,000 deaths among 75,000 women. *Lancet* 1992; 339: 1 15, 71–85.
5 Stewart LA, Pignon JP, Arriagada R, Souhami RI, on behalf of the NSCLC Collaborative Group. A meta-analysis using individual patient data from randomised clinical trials of chemotherapy in non-small cell lung cancer. I. Survival in the surgical setting [abstract]. *Proceedings of the American Society of Clinical Oncology* 1994; 13: 336.
6 Stewart LA, Parmar MKB. Meta-analysis of the literature or of individual patient data: is there a difference? *Lancet* 1993; 341: 418–22.
7 Pignon JP, Arriagada R. Meta-analysis. *Lancet* 1993; 341: 964–5.
8 Dickersin K, Scherer R, Lefebvre C. Identification of relevant studies for systematic reviews. *BMJ* 1994; 309: 1286–91. (Chapter 3)
9 Simes J. Publication bias; the case for an international registry of clinical trials. *J Clin Oncol* 1986; 4: 1529–41.
10 Gregory WM, Richards MA, Malpas JS. Combination chemotherapy versus melphalan and prednisolone in the treatment of multiple myeloma: an overview of published trials. *J Clin Oncol* 1992; 10: 334–42.
11 Advanced Ovarian Cancer Trialists' Group. Chemotherapy in advanced ovarian cancer: an overview of randomised clinical trials. *BMJ* 1991; 303: 884–9.
12 Peto R, Pike M, Armitage P, Breslow NE, Cox DR, Howard SV, et al. Design and analysis of randomised clinical trials requiring prolonged observation of each patient. I. Introduction and design. *Br J Cancer* 1976; 34: 585–612.
13 Hoover HC, Brandhorst JS, Peters LC, Surdyke MG, Takeshita Y, Madariaga J, et al. Adjuvant active specific immunotherapy for human colorectal cancer: 6·5 year median follow-up of a phase II prospectively randomised trial. *J Clin Oncol* 1993; 11: 390–9.
14 Hoover HC, Surdyke MG, Dangel RB, Peters LC, Hanna MG. Prospectively randomised trial of adjuvant active-specific immunotherapy for human colorectal cancer. *Cancer* 1985; 55: 1236–43.
15 What's wrong with the BMJ? [editor's choice]. *BMJ* 1994 January 8, 308: i.

# 5 Why sources of heterogeneity in meta-analysis should be investigated

SIMON G THOMPSON

## Summary

Although meta-analysis is now well established as a method of combining the results of separate but similar studies, an uncritical use of the technique can be very misleading. One common problem is the failure to investigate appropriately the sources of heterogeneity, in particular the clinical differences between the studies included. This paper distinguishes between the concepts of clinical and statistical heterogeneity and exemplifies the importance of investigating heterogeneity by using published meta-analyses of epidemiological studies of serum cholesterol concentration and clinical trials of its reduction. Although not without some dangers of speculative conclusions, prompted by overzealous inspection of the data to hand, a sensible investigation of sources of heterogeneity should increase the relevance of the results of meta-analyses.

The purpose of a meta-analysis of a set of clinical trials is rather different from the specific aims of an individual trial. For example, a particular clinical trial investigating the effect of serum cholesterol reduction on the risk of ischaemic heart disease tests a particular treatment regimen, given for a specified duration to participants fulfilling certain selection criteria, using a particular definition of outcome measures. The purpose of a meta-analysis of cholesterol lowering trials is broader—that is, to estimate the extent to which serum cholesterol reduction, achieved by a variety of means, generally influences the risk of ischaemic heart disease. A meta-analysis also attempts to gain greater objectivity, generalisability, and precision by including all the available evidence from randomised trials that pertain to the issue.[1] Because of the broader aims of a meta-analysis, the trials included usually encompass a substantial variety of specific treatment regimens, types of patients, and outcomes. In this chapter I argue that the influence of these clinical differences between trials, or clinical heterogeneity, on the overall results needs to be explored carefully.

I start by clarifying the relation between clinical heterogeneity and statistical heterogeneity. I then give examples of meta-analyses of both observational epidemiological studies of serum cholesterol concentration and clinical trials of its reduction in which exploration of heterogeneity was important in the overall conclusions reached. The discussion addresses the dangers of post hoc exploration of results and consequent overinterpretation.

## Clinical and statistical heterogeneity

To make the concepts clear, it is useful to focus on a meta-analysis where heterogeneity was found to be a problem in its interpretation. Figure 5.1 shows the results of 19 randomised trials investigating the use of endoscopic sclerotherapy for reducing mortality in the primary treatment of cirrhotic patients with oesophageal varices.[2] As is usual, the results of each trial are shown as odds ratios and 95% confidence intervals, with odds ratios less than unity representing a beneficial effect of sclerotherapy. As is noted in the original paper, the trials differed considerably in their patient selection, baseline disease severity, endoscopic technique, management of intermediate outcomes such as variceal bleeding, and duration of follow up.[2] So in this meta-analysis, as in almost all, there is extensive clinical heterogeneity. There were also methodological differences in the

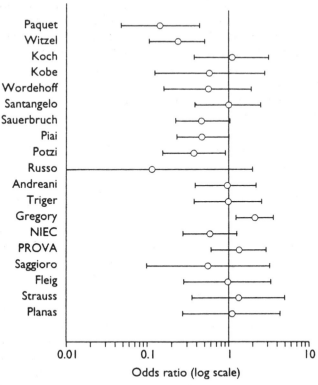

Figure 5.1 Odds ratios of death (and 95% confidence intervals) in 19 trials of sclerotherapy. Odds ratios less than unity represent beneficial effects of sclerotherapy. Trials are identified by principal author, referenced by Pagliaro et al[2]

mechanism of randomisation and in the extent and handling of withdrawals and losses to follow up.

It would not be surprising, therefore, to find that the results of these trials were to some degree incompatible with one another. Such incompatibility in the quantitative results is termed statistical heterogeneity. Statistical heterogencity may be caused by known clinical differences between trials or by methodological differences, or it may be related to unknown or unrecorded trial characteristics. In assessing the direct evidence of statistical heterogeneity, the imprecision in the estimate of the odds ratio for each trial, as expressed by the confidence interval in figure 5.1, has to be taken into account. The statistical question is then whether there is greater variation between the results of the trials than is compatible with the play of chance. As might be surmised from inspection of figure 5.1, the published test of statistical heterogeneity yielded a highly significant result ($\chi^2_{18} = 43$, $P < 0.001$), giving very substantial evidence of statistical heterogeneity.[2] (For the interpretation of such tests, it is useful to know that a $\chi^2$ statistic has on average a value equal to its degrees of freedom, so a result of $\chi^2_{18} = 18.0$ would give no evidence of heterogeneity; values much larger, such as that observed for the sclerotherapy trials, give small P values and provide evidence of statistical heterogeneity.)

The existence of clinical heterogeneity would be expected to lead to at least some degree of statistical heterogeneity in the results. In the example of the sclerotherapy trials, the evidence for statistical heterogeneity is substantial. In many meta-analyses, however, statistical evidence for heterogeneity will be lacking and the test of heterogeneity will be non-significant. Yet this cannot be interpreted as evidence of homogeneity (that is, total consistency) of the results of all the trials included. This is not only because a non-significant test can never be interpreted as direct evidence in favour of the null hypothesis (of total consistency),[3] but in particular because such tests of heterogeneity have low power and may fail to detect as statistically significant even a moderate degree of genuine heterogeneity.[4] [5]

We would of course be somewhat happier to ignore the problems of clinical heterogeneity in the interpretation of the results if direct evidence of statistical heterogeneity is lacking, and more inclined to try to understand the reasons for any heterogeneity for which the evidence is more convincing. However, the extent of statistical heterogeneity, which can be quantified,[6] is more important than the evidence of its existence. The guiding principle should be to investigate the influences of the specific clinical differences between studies rather than to rely on an overall statistical test of heterogeneity. This then focuses attention on particular contrasts between the trials included, which will be more powerful at detecting genuine differences—and more relevant to the overall conclusions. For example, in the sclerotherapy trials, the underlying disease severity as evidenced by the rate of bleeding varices was discussed as being potentially related to the efficacy of sclerotherapy observed.[2]

The most important conclusion of a meta-analysis is usually the quantitative summary of the results—for example, in terms of an overall odds ratio and 95% confidence interval. For the sclerotherapy trials, the overall odds ratio for death was given as 0·76 with a 95% confidence interval of 0·61 to 0·94.[2] A naive interpretation of this would be that sclerotherapy convincingly decreased the risk of death, with an odds reduction of around 25%. But what are the implications of clinical and statistical heterogeneity in the interpretation of this result? Given the clinical heterogeneity, we do not know to which endoscopic technique, to which selection of patients, or in conjunction with what ancillary clinical management such a conclusion is supposed to refer. It is some sort of "average" statement that is not easy to interpret quantitatively in relation to the benefits that might accrue from the use of a specific clinical protocol. In this particular case the evidence for statistical heterogeneity is also overwhelming and this, as stated in the original meta-analysis,[2] introduces even more doubt about the interpretation of any one overall estimate of effect. Even if we accept that some sort of average or typical[7] effect is being estimated, the confidence interval given is too narrow in terms of extrapolating the results to future trials or patients, since the extra variability between the results of the different trials is ignored.[5]

The answer to such problems is that meta-analyses should incorporate a careful investigation of potential sources of heterogeneity. Three examples of the benefits of applying such an approach in published meta-analyses are now given. An obvious example is provided by the relation of serum cholesterol concentration and the risk of ischaemic heart disease in prospective studies; a more challenging example is the relation of a reduction in serum cholesterol to the risk of ischaemic heart disease in clinical trials; and a more speculative example is the relation of serum cholesterol concentration to the risk of cancer.

## Serum cholesterol concentration and risk of ischaemic heart disease

An extreme example of heterogeneity is evident in a recent review of the 10 largest prospective studies of serum cholesterol concentration and the risk of ischaemic heart disease in men, which included data on 19 000 myocardial infarctions or deaths

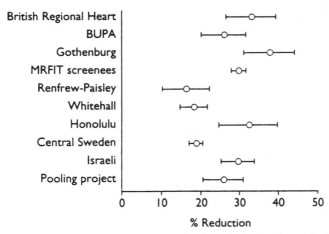

Figure 5.2 Percentage reduction in risk of ischaemic heart disease (and 95% confidence intervals) associated with 0·6 mmol/l serum cholesterol reduction in 10 prospective studies of men. Studies referenced by Law et al[8]

from ischaemic heart disease.[8] Here the purpose was to summarise the magnitude of the relation between serum cholesterol and risk of ischaemic heart disease in order to estimate the long term benefit that might be expected to accrue from reduction in serum cholesterol concentrations.

Figure 5.2 shows the results from the prospective studies. These are expressed as proportionate reductions in risk associated with a reduction in serum cholesterol of 0·6 mmol/l (about 10% of average levels in Western countries), having been derived from the apparently log-linear associations of risk of ischaemic heart disease with serum cholesterol concentration. They also take into account the underestimation of the relation of risk of ischaemic heart disease that results from the fact that a single measurement of serum cholesterol is an imprecise estimate of long term level, sometimes termed regression dilution bias.[9] Although all of the 10 studies showed that cholesterol reduction was associated with a reduction in the risk of ischaemic heart disease, they differed substantially in the estimated magnitude of this effect. This is clear from figure 5.2, and an extreme value for an overall test of heterogeneity ($\chi_9^2 = 127$, P $<<$ 0·001) is obtained. This shows that simply combining the results of these studies into one overall estimate is misleading; an understanding of the reasons for the heterogeneity is necessary.

The most obvious cause of the heterogeneity relates to the ages of the participants, or more particularly the average age of experiencing coronary events during follow up, since it is well known that the relative risk of ischaemic heart disease with a given serum cholesterol increment declines with advancing age.[10] [11] The data from the 10 studies were therefore divided, as far as was possible from published and unpublished information, into groups according to age at entry.[8] This yielded 26 substudies, the results of which were plotted against the average age of experiencing a coronary event (fig 5.3). The percentage reduction in ischaemic heart disease clearly decreases with age. This relation could be summarised with a quadratic regression on age, appropriately weighted to take account of the different precisions of each estimate. It was concluded that a decrease in cholesterol concentration of 0·6 mmol/l was associated with a decrease in risk of ischaemic heart disease of 54% at age 40, 39% at age 50, 27% at age 60, 20% at age 70, and 19% at age 80. In fact, there remains considerable evidence of heterogeneity in figure 5.3 even from this summary of results ($\chi^2_{23} = 45$, $P = 0·005$), but it is far less extreme than the heterogeneity evident before age was considered (fig 5.2).

The effect of the conclusions brought about by considering age are of course crucial—for example, in considering the impact of cholesterol reduction in the population. The proportionate

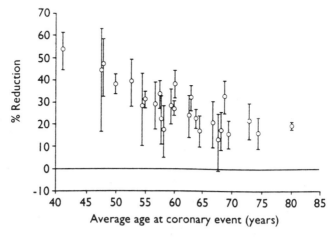

Figure 5.3 Percentage reduction in risk of ischaemic heart disease (and 95% confidence intervals) associated with 0·6 mmol/l serum cholesterol reduction, according to age at experiencing a coronary event

reductions in the risk of ischaemic heart disease associated with reduction in serum cholesterol are strongly related to age. The large proportionate reductions in early middle age cannot be extrapolated to old ages, at which more modest proportionate reductions are evident.

## Serum cholesterol reduction and risk of ischaemic heart disease

The randomised controlled trials of serum cholesterol reduction have been the subject of a number of recent meta-analyses[8] [12] [13] and much controversy. In conjunction with the review of the 10 prospective studies just described, the results of 28 randomised trials were summarised in order to quantify the observed effect of serum cholesterol reduction on the risk of ischaemic heart disease in the short term, the trials having an average duration of about five years.[8] There was considerable clinical heterogeneity between the trials in the interventions tested (different drugs, different diets, and in one case surgical intervention using partial ileal bypass grafting), in the duration of the trials (0·3 to 10 years), in the average extent of serum cholesterol reduction achieved (0·3 to 1·5 mmol/l), and in the selection criteria for the patients such as pre-existing disease (for example, primary or secondary prevention trials) and level of serum cholesterol concentration at entry. As before it would seem likely that these substantial clinical differences would lead to some heterogeneity in the observed results.

Conventional meta-analysis diagrams such as figure 5.1 are not very useful for investigating heterogeneity. A better diagram for this purpose was proposed by Galbraith[14] and is shown for the risk of ischaemic heart disease in figure 5.4. For each trial the ratio of the log odds ratio to its standard error (the Z statistic) is plotted against the reciprocal of the standard error. Hence the least precise results from small trials appear towards the left of the figure and results from the largest trials appear towards the right. An overall (log) odds ratio is represented by the slope of the solid line through the origin in the figure. The dotted lines are positioned two units above and below the solid line and delimit an area in which, in the absence of statistical heterogeneity, the great majority (that is, about 95%) of the trial results would be

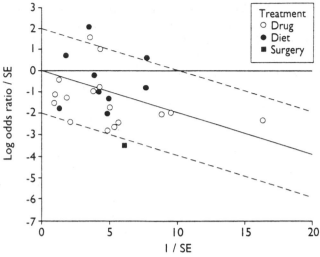

Figure 5.4 Galbraith plot of odds ratios of ischaemic heart disease in 28 trials of serum cholesterol reduction (see text for explanation). Two trials were omitted because of no events in one group

expected to lie. It is thus interesting to note the characteristics of those trials that lie near or outside these dotted lines. For example, in figure 5.4 there are two dietary trials that lie above the upper line and showed apparently adverse effects of serum

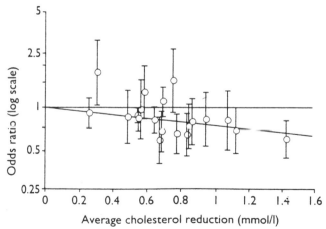

Figure 5.5 Odds ratios of ischaemic heart disease (and 95% confidence intervals) according to the average extent of serum cholesterol reduction achieved in each of 28 trials. Overall summary of results is indicated by sloping line. Results of the nine smallest trials have been combined

cholesterol reduction on the risk of ischaemic heart disease. One of these trials achieved only a very small cholesterol reduction; the other had a particularly short duration.[15] Conversely the surgical trial, below the bottom dotted line and showing a large reduction in the risk of ischaemic heart disease, was both the longest trial and the one that achieved the greatest cholesterol reduction.[15] These observations add weight to the need to investigate heterogeneity of results according to extent and duration of cholesterol reduction.

Figure 5.5 shows the results according to average extent of cholesterol reduction achieved. There is very strong evidence (P < 0·001) that the proportionate reduction in the risk of ischaemic heart disease increases with the extent of average cholesterol reduction.[15] A suitable summary of the trial results, represented by the sloping line in figure 5.5, is that the risk of ischaemic heart disease is reduced by an estimated 18% (95% confidence interval 13% to 22%) for each 0·6 mmol/l reduction in serum cholesterol concentration. Obtaining data subdivided by time since randomisation[8] to investigate the effect of duration was

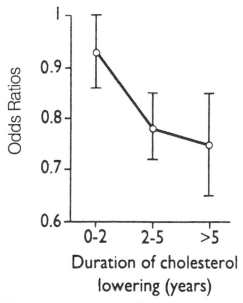

Figure 5.6 Odds ratios of ischaemic heart disease (and 95% confidence intervals) per 0.6 mmol/l serum cholesterol reduction in 28 trials, according to the duration of cholesterol lowering

also very informative (fig 5.6). Whereas the reduction in ischaemic heart disease risk in the first two years was rather limited, the reductions thereafter were around 25% per 0·6 mmol/l reduction. After extent and duration of cholesterol reduction were allowed for in this way, the evidence for further heterogeneity of the results from the differential trials was limited (P = 0·11). In particular there was no evidence of further differences in the results between the drug and the dietary trials or between the primary prevention and the secondary prevention trials.[8] [15]

This investigation of heterogeneity was also crucial to the conclusions reached. The analysis showed that the percentage reduction in the risk of ischaemic heart disease depends on the extent and duration of cholesterol reduction. Meta-analyses ignoring these factors[12] [13] may well be misleading. It also seems that these factors are more important determinants of the proportionate reduction in ischaemic heart disease than the mode of intervention or the underlying risk of the patient. Patients at high risk of ischaemic heart disease of course have most to gain from cholesterol reduction in absolute terms for ischaemic heart disease and in both proportionate and absolute terms for all cause mortality.[12] Investigation of treatment benefits according to the underlying risk of the patient is one particular aspect of heterogeneity.[16] However, analyses that simply relate the event rate in the treated group (or the odds ratio of treated subjects to controls) to the event rate in the control group—using regression, for example—need very careful interpretation because of the problems induced by regression to the mean.[17]

## Serum cholesterol concentration and the risk of cancer

An association between low serum cholesterol concentrations and increased risk of cancer has been identified in a number of epidemiological prospective studies, and in 1991 a meta-analysis of the results from the 33 available prospective studies was published.[18] Because preclinical cancer is associated with low serum cholesterol, attention focused on cancers diagnosed at least two years and cancer deaths occurring at least five years after cholesterol measurement. Here these results for men (table 5.1) are discussed. The relation between cancer risk and serum cholesterol was summarised as the mean cholesterol in those subsequently developing cancer minus the mean in those who did not. Hence a negative mean difference in cholesterol corresponds to an association of low cholesterol levels with an increased risk of cancer. The overall mean difference for all the 33 studies was indeed negative, $-0.04$ mmol/l in table 5.1. This is significant ($P < 0.001$) but small, being equivalent to about a 15% increase in the lowest fifth of the distribution of cholesterol levels relative to all the remainder of the distribution. Of interest here is that there was some evidence of statistical heterogeneity between the results of the different studies ($\chi^2_{32} = 53$, $P = 0.01$; table 5.1).

Investigation of possible sources of heterogeneity revealed that the predominant socioeconomic status of the men recruited seemed to be important (table 5.1). The association between low cholesterol and increased risk of cancer seemed most pronounced in studies of men with predominantly low socioeconomic status, moderate in studies of mixed populations, and absent or even reversed in the studies of men with high socioeconomic status. After this division of studies according to socioeconomic status, the heterogeneity was substantially less ($\chi^2_{30} = 37$, $P = 0.18$). Thus socioeconomic grouping seemed to explain a substantial part of the original heterogeneity of results.

Table 5.1 *Prospective studies of serum cholesterol concentration and the risk of cancer in men*[18]: *cancers diagnosed at least two years and cancer deaths occurring at least five years after cholesterol measurement*

| | No of cancer cases | No of studies | Mean (SE) difference in serum cholesterol (mmol/l)* | Heterogeneity |
|---|---|---|---|---|
| All studies: | | | | |
| Overall | 12 516 | 33 | $-0.041$ (0.009) | $\chi^2 = 53$, df $= 32$, $P = 0.01$ |
| Socioeconomic status: | | | | |
| High | 619 | 4 | $+0.032$ (0.048) | |
| Mixed | 10 378 | 20 | $-0.030$ (0.010) | $\chi^2 = 37$, df $= 30$, $P = 0.18$ |
| Low | 1 519 | 9 | $-0.130$ (0.025) | |
| Studies with lung cancer data: | | | | |
| All cancers | 8 062 | 19 | $-0.043$ (0.012) | $\chi^2 = 40$, df $= 18$, $P = 0.002$ |
| Lung cancers | 2 239 | 19 | $-0.101$ (0.022) | $\chi^2 = 36$, df $= 18$, $P = 0.007$ |
| Cancers other than lung | 5 823 | 19 | $-0.023$ (0.014) | $\chi^2 = 32$, df $= 18$, $P = 0.02$ |

* Mean cholesterol in those who subsequently developed cancers minus mean in those who did not.

Another subdivision considered was that according to cancer site. Where data were available, results within studies were separated into lung cancers and other cancers (table 5.1). Lung cancers accounted for most of the overall association with serum cholesterol concentration and showed similar heterogeneity according to socioeconomic status as described above. The association for other cancers was less statistically significant, and showed less evidence of heterogeneity. This suggests that a factor particularly related to lung cancer, presumably cigarette smoking, is involved in the explanation of these results.

Although there may be other explanations, these findings with respect to socioeconomic status and lung cancer suggest an explanation in terms of confounding by the intensity of cigarette smoking.[18] For example, more intensive smoking among poorer people who may have lower serum cholesterol concentrations could produce the observed results. Such an explanation requires confirmation, but the heterogeneity is important in that it tends to argue against a conclusion that low cholesterol concentrations are a direct cause of cancer.

## Discussion

As meta-analysis becomes widely used as a technique for synthesizing the results of separate primary studies, an overly simplistic approach to its implementation needs to be avoided. A failure to investigate potential sources of clinical heterogeneity is one aspect of this. As shown in the above examples, such investigation can importantly affect the overall conclusions to be drawn, as well as the clinical implications of the review. Therefore the issues of clinical and statistical heterogeneity and how to approach them need emphasis in written guidelines and in the computer software currently being developed for conducting meta-analyses.[19]

Discussion of heterogeneity in meta-analysis affects whether it is reasonable to believe in one overall estimate that applies to all the studies encompassed, implied by the so called fixed effect method of statistical analysis.[3] Undue reliance may have been put on this approach in the past, causing overly simplistic and overly dogmatic interpretation.[5] Although the so called random effects method of analysis[6] may be useful when statistical heterogeneity is present but cannot be obviously explained by clinical differences, the main focus should be on trying to understand any sources of heterogeneity that are present. In practice, however, there may be no great difference between those who advocate a fixed effect approach[7] and those who are more doubtful[5 20 21] when it comes to undertaking particular meta-analyses. For example, the recent large scale overview of early breast cancer treatment, carried out ostensibly with a fixed effect approach, includes an appropriate investigation of heterogeneity according to type and duration of treatment, dose of drug, use of concomitant therapy, age, nodal status, oestrogen receptor status, and outcome (recurrence or death).[22] Likewise, extensive investigation of heterogeneity was undertaken in the recent overview of antiplatelet therapy.[23]

Considerable dangers of overinterpretation can, however, be induced by attempting to investigate heterogeneity, since such investigations are usually inspired, at least to some extent, by looking at the results to hand. Moreover, apparent (even statistically significant) heterogeneity may always be due to chance, and search for its cause would then be misleading. The problem is akin to that of subgroup analyses within an individual clinical trial.[24] However the degree of clinical heterogeneity across different clinical trials is greater than that within individual trials and represents a more serious problem. Guidelines for deciding whether to believe results that stem from investigation of heterogeneity depend on, for example, the magnitude and statistical significance of the differences identified, the extent to which the potential sources of heterogeneity had been specified in advance, and indirect evidence and biological considerations which support the investigation.[25]

These problems in meta-analysis are greatest when there are many clinical differences but only a small number of trials available. In such situations there may be several alternative explanations of statistical heterogeneity, and ideas about sources of heterogeneity can be considered only as hypotheses for evaluation in future studies. Some of these problems may be more satisfactorily approached by basing meta-analyses on the individual patient data from each trial[26] rather than their summary results (see chapter 4), so that divisions according to patients' characteristics can be made within trials and these results combined across trials.

Although I have focused on clinical causes of heterogeneity, it is important to recognise that there are other potential causes. Statistical heterogeneity may be caused by publication bias[27] (in that among small trials those with dramatic results may be preferentially published), by defects of methodological quality,[28] or even by early termination of clinical trials for ethical reasons.[29] For example, poor methodological quality was of concern in the meta-analysis of sclerotherapy trials discussed at the beginning of this chapter. Statistical heterogeneity may also be induced by using an inappropriate scale for measuring treatment effects—for example, using absolute rather than relative differences.

Despite the laudable attempts to achieve objectivity in reviewing scientific data, considerable subjective judgment is necessary in deciding whether and how to use meta-analysis. These judgments include those about which studies are "relevant" and which studies are methodologically sound enough to be included in a statistical synthesis, as well as the issue of whether and how to investigate sources of heterogeneity. Such scientific judgments are as necessary in meta-analysis as they are in other forms of medical research, and skills in recognising appropriate analyses and dismissing overly speculative interpretations need to be developed. However, in many meta-analyses heterogeneity can and should be investigated so as to increase the clinical relevance of the conclusions drawn and the scientific understanding of the studies reviewed.

I thank Peter England and Rebecca Hardy for their constructive criticisms of a previous version of this chapter.

1 Dickersin K, Berlin J. Meta-analysis: state-of-the-science. *Epidemiol Rev* 1992; 14: 154–76.

2 Pagliaro L, D'Amico G, Sorensen TIA, Lebrec D, Burroughs AK, Morabito A, *et al*. Prevention of first bleeding in cirrhosis: a meta-analysis of randomised trials of non-surgical treatment. *Ann Intern Med* 1992; 117: 59–70.

3 Altman DG. *Practical statistics for medical research*. London: Chapman and Hall, 1991: 167–70.

4 Whitehead A, Whitehead J. A general parametric approach to the meta-analysis of randomised clinical trials. *Stat Med* 1991; 10: 1665–77.

5 Thompson SG, Pocock SJ. Can meta-analyses be trusted? *Lancet* 1991; 338: 1127–30.

6 DerSimonian R, Laird N. Meta-analysis in clinical trials. *Controlled Clin Trials* 1986; 7: 177–88.

7 Peto R. Why do we need systematic overviews of randomised trials? *Stat Med* 1987; 6: 233–40.

8 Law MR, Wald NJ, Thompson SG. By how much and how quickly does reduction in serum cholesterol concentration lower risk of ischaemic heart disease? *BMJ* 1994; 308: 367–73.

9 MacMahon S, Peto R, Cutler J, Collins R, Sorlie P, Neaton J, *et al*. Blood pressure, stroke, and coronary heart disease. Part I, prolonged differences in blood pressure: prospective observational studies corrected for the regression dilution bias. *Lancet* 1990; 335: 765–74.

10 Manolio TA, Pearson TA, Wenger NK, Barrett-Connor E, Payne GH, Harlan WR.

Cholesterol and heart disease in older persons and women: review of an NHLBI workshop. *Ann Epidemiol* 1992; **2**: 161–76.

11 Shipley MJ, Pocock SJ, Marmot MG. Does plasma cholesterol concentration predict mortality from coronary heart disease in elderly people? 18 year follow-up in Whitehall study. *BMJ* 1991; **303**: 89–92.

12 Ravnskov U. Cholesterol lowering trials in coronary heart disease: frequency of citation and outcome. *BMJ* 1992; **305**: 15–19.

13 Davey Smith G, Song F, Sheldon T. Cholesterol lowering and mortality: the importance of considering initial level of risk. *BMJ* 1993; **306**: 1376–73.

14 Galbraith RF. A note on the graphical presentation of estimated odds ratios from several clinical trials. *Stat Med* 1988; **7**: 889–94.

15 Thompson SG. Controversies in meta-analysis: the case of the trials of serum cholesterol reduction. *Stat Meth Med Res* 1993; **2**: 173–92.

16 Brand R, Kragt H. Importance of trends in the interpretation of an overall odds ratio in the meta-analysis of clinical trials. *Stat Med* 1992; **11**: 2077–82.

17 Senn S. Importance of trends in the interpretation of an overall odds ratio in a meta-analysis of clinical trials. *Stat Med* 1994; **13**: 293–6.

18 Law MR, Thompson SG. Low serum cholesterol and the risk of cancer: an analysis of the published prospective studies. *Cancer Causes Control* 1991; **2**: 253–61.

19 Oxman A. Preparing and maintaining systematic reviews. In: Sackett D, ed. *Cochrane Collaboration Handbook*. Section VI. Oxford: Cochrane Collaboration, 1994.

20 Meier P. Meta-analysis of clinical trials as a scientific discipline [commentary]. *Stat Med* 1987; **6**: 329–31.

21 Bailey KR. Inter-study differences: how should they influence the interpretation and analysis of results? *Stat Med* 1987; **6**: 351–8.

22 Early Breast Cancer Trialists' Collaborative Group. Systemic treatment of early breast cancer by hormonal, cytotoxic, or immune therapy. *Lancet* 1992; **339**: 1–15, 71–85.

23 Antiplatelet Trialists' Collaboration. Collaborative overview of randomised trials of antiplatelet therapy. I. Prevention of death, myocardial infarction, and stroke by prolonged antiplatelet therapy in various categories of patients. *BMJ* 1994; **308**: 81–106.

24 Yusuf S, Wittes J, Probstfield J, Tyroler HA. Analysis and interpretation of treatment effects in subgroups of patients in randomised clinical trials. *JAMA* 1991; **266**: 93–8.

25 Oxman AD, Guyatt GH. A consumer's guide to subgroup analyses. *Ann Intern Med* 1992; **116**: 78–84.

26 Stewart LA, Parmar MKB. Meta-analysis of the literature or of individual patient data: is there a difference? *Lancet* 1993; **341**: 418–22.

27 Easterbrook PJ, Berlin JA, Gopalan R, Matthews DR. Publication bias in clinical research. *Lancet* 1991; **337**: 867–72.

28 Schulz KF, Chalmers I, Hayes RJ, Altman DG. Empirical evidence of bias: dimensions of methodological quality are associated with estimates of treatment effects. *JAMA* 1995; **273**: 408–12.

29 Hughes MD, Freedman LS, Pocock SJ. The impact of stopping rules on heterogeneity of results in overviews of clinical trials. *Biometrics* 1992; **48**: 41–53.

# 6 Problems with meta-analysis

H J EYSENCK

## Summary

Including all relevant material—good, bad, and indifferent—in a meta-analysis delegates to the reader the subjective judgments that meta-analysis was designed to avoid. Several problems arise in meta-analysis: regressions are often non-linear; effects are often multivariate rather than univariate; coverage can be restricted; bad studies may be included; the data summarised may not be homogeneous; grouping different causal factors may lead to meaningless estimated effect sizes; and the failure to relate data to theories may obscure discrepancies. Meta-analysis may often not be the one best method for studying the diversity of fields for which it has been used.

Why do we undertake systematic reviews of a given field? The most important reason is perhaps that we are concerned about a particular theory and wish to know how the evidence for and against stacks up. There are also practical reasons; single studies often use small numbers of participants, and basing our estimates of effect sizes on large numbers of studies drastically narrows the confidence interval around our estimates. Traditional reviews are often not very systematic, and are frequently biased. Systematic reviews can be of several different kinds: meta-analyses, including (we hope) all relevant material, good, bad, and indifferent, and leading to an estimate of effect size;[1-3] best-evidence synthesis;[4] and the hypothetico-deductive approach,[5] in which the effort is directed at evaluating the evidence for and against a given theory, in an attempt to solve the problem of why contradictory results appear, rather than simply averaging often incompatible data.

## Inclusiveness of meta-analysis

Critics may object to my statement that meta-analysis involves material, good, bad, and indifferent, but consider the study by Smith *et al* (discussed in more detail later), which numbered among its authors the originator of the term.[6] The authors complained about the subjectivity that had led previous reviewers of studies assessing the effects of psychotherapy to exclude certain studies because of alleged design faults. This is what they claim to have done to overcome this subjectivity: "the method used is called meta-analysis. It is the statistical summary of the numerical outcomes of each study. We attempted to find and include all the controlled studies of psychotherapy outcome; that is, all the research in which one group of persons was treated for psychological conditions and compared with another, roughly equivalent untreated group. Studies were not excluded from consideration on arbitrary grounds; for example, because they used relatively inexperienced therapists or clients who had volunteered for the experiment, or had crude outcome measures. We suspected that contradictory conclusions of previous reviewers were largely the result of the arbitrary imposition of criteria for deciding which studies constituted valid evidence. These criteria had often been applied so as to favour a favourite hypothesis or vested ideological interest."

In other words, the crucial feature of this study was a statistical summary of the results of all relevant studies, however bad; indeed, later on the authors compared the results of what they considered good and bad studies, demonstrating that they were aware that many of the studies included were subject to damaging criticism. As noted by Knipschild in chapter 2, "it does not make sense to combine the top [best] with the other [not so good articles] and do a statistical precision . . . meta-analysis."[7]

A good review is based on intimate personal knowledge of the field, the participants, the problems that arise, the reputation of different laboratories, the likely trustworthiness of individual scientists, and other partly subjective but extremely relevant considerations. Meta-analysis ignores such subjective factors. It can be done by simply feeding the published results to a computer and coming up with an effect size. The computer avoids the bias of the subjective approach but simply adds together the biases of the authors of the original reports—which may or may not balance out.

I have pointed out problems that arise in the use of meta-analysis[5 8 9]; although the same problems may arise in connection with other methods of systematic reviewing, they are particularly likely to apply to meta-analysis. Let me list the problems that arise in this mechanical process.

## Problems of meta-analytical process

### Regressions are often non-linear

Glass and Smith carried out a meta-analysis of research on class size and achievement and concluded that "a clear and strong relationship between class size and achievement has emerged."[10] The study was done and analysed well; it might almost be cited as an example of what meta-analysis can do. Yet the conclusion is very misleading, as is the estimate of effect size it presents: "between class-size of 40 pupils and one pupil lie more than 30 percentile ranks of achievement." Such estimates imply a linear regression, yet the regression is extremely curvilinear, as one of the authors' figures shows: between class sizes of 20 and 40 there is absolutely no difference in achievement; it is only with unusually small classes that there seems to be an effect. For a teacher the major result is that for 90% of all classes the number of pupils makes no difference at all to their achievement. The conclusions drawn by the authors from their meta-analysis are formally correct, but they are statistically meaningless and particularly misleading. No estimate of effect size is meaningful unless regressions are linear, yet such linearity is seldom investigated, or, if not present, taken seriously. A simple traditional review would not have made such an obvious error.

### Effects are often multivariate rather than univariate

Consider the effect of passive smoking on lung cancer, where several meta-analyses (and best evidence analyses) have been conducted[11-13]; these all assume a univariate relation, although they come to quite disparate conclusions. Now consider the work of Janerich *et al*, who carried out a well planned study of the effects of passive smoking on lung cancer, and concluded that "the evidence we report lends further support to the observation that passive smoking may increase the risk of subsequent lung cancer."[14] In this study, individually matched pairs (lung cancer patients and healthy controls) were compared for exposure to cigarette smoke in four different situations. For overall exposure, "no clear dose-response relationship is evident," suggesting no overall effect. For exposure in childhood and adolescence there is an overall effect. For smoking by the spouse, the most widely used measure, "there was little evidence of a trend according to amount of exposure." Exposure in the workplace indicated "no evidence of an adverse effect of environmental tobacco smoke." Finally, "our analysis of exposure in social settings . . . showed a statistically significant inverse association between environmental tobacco smoke and lung cancer."

What would a proper summary of this work be? It would emphasise the lack of overall effects, showing no clear dose-response relation; the negative health effects of childhood and adolescent passive smoking would be contrasted with the positive health effects of smoking in social situations; and the summary would also include the lack of any detected effect of workplace or spouse smoking. The authors concentrate on the one result out of four that is negatively significant, forgetting that statistical significance for one selected test out of four cannot be calculated as if this were the only test done (there was no Bonferroni correction), and attempt to explain it by suggesting that during childhood and adolescence probands are more likely to be responsive to passive smoking, although "we know of no specific mechanism that would explain our findings." In other words, the explanation is purely ad hoc and adds nothing to the alleged findings. The authors fail to discuss the fact that "the difference in the magnitude of the effect between exposure during childhood and adolescence and exposure during adulthood did not achieve statistical significance," a finding that would seem to disprove their own hypothesis.

Can the "unexpected" protective effect of exposure to social smoking be explained? A likely hypothesis would suggest that extraverted personality traits seem to protect against cancer and that individuals prone to cancer have personality traits usually associated with introversion.[15] Extraverted people, however, are more likely than introverted ones to attend social functions and to be exposed to cigarette smoke there. The hypotheses would explain the alleged protective function of social smoking as an artefact; such protection is due to personality characteristics shared by socially active people and people not prone to cancer. The failure of Janerich et al to take into account any risk factors other than smoking accounts for the failure to explain their own findings. The positive relation between environmental tobacco smoke and lung cancer in childhood may be due to genetic factors linking parents and children.[15]

Looking at this study from the point of view of simple meta-analysis, or even best evidence summary, we would simply note an overall failure of environmental tobacco smoke to be linked with lung cancer. The hypothetico-deductive approach, however, would single out the obvious contradiction between results for social smoking and smoking in childhood, try to explain them, and suggest that in further research factors like personality and genetics should be taken into account. Indeed, these factors have been shown to be important in the effects of smoking, and no study leaving out a consideration of genetics, personality, stress, etc, is worth summarising in a meta-analysis, or any other type of analysis, because it attempts a univariate type of analysis of a clearly multivariate problem.[15]

### Restriction of coverage

Meta-analysis always specifies the nature of the material to be included; in the case of passive smoking and health this would normally be studies comparing health records of individuals exposed or not exposed to passive smoking and suffering or not suffering from various diseases believed to be related to smoking. This enables us to obtain an estimate of the size of putative effects of exposure. Looking at the problem from the point of the hypothetico-deductive methodology, however, such a procedure leaves out vitally relevant evidence. I will give an example. Lee carried out a meta-analysis on about 100 studies in an effort to discover the extent of misclassification when smokers pretend to be non-smokers.[16] He found that in smoking cessation studies, percentages in excess of 15-20% were commonplace, ranging up to 40% of misclassified non-smokers. Again, the percentage of true smokers found among self reported non-smokers tended to be higher in studies of men and women with lung cancer than in studies of those without lung cancer. In general, Lee suggests that of self reported never smokers, 2·5% arc actually current smokers and 10% have smoked in the past. These figures may seem to suggest a rather modest level of deception, but it is sufficient to cause Lee to conclude "that the epidemiologically observed association between passive smoking and lung cancer arose from bias due to misclassification of a proportion of smokers as non-smokers."

Clearly this suggestion is of vital relevance to any consideration of the theory that passive smoking causes (or is related to) lung cancer, yet the meta-analyses of this topic quoted always failed to consider it because the structure of meta-analysis is concerned with estimates of the size and significance of effect but not with the possible causes of the observed effect, which are always interpreted in terms of the original hypotheses involved without looking at evidence suggesting alternative interpretations. It is of course open to the investigator to step outside the rigid limitations of the meta-analysis format and add a discussion of alternative interpretations of the observed effect size, but this is strictly outside the rules imposed by meta-analysis and forms no part of its raison d'être.

### Quality of studies

Some proponents of meta-analysis pride themselves on the inclusiveness of the method, rejecting the notion that bad studies should be excluded as "subjective." Yet such evaluation is part and parcel of the special insight which the expert can bring to the discussion, and inclusion of bad studies may completely subvert the true outcome of a hypothetico-deductive analysis. Consider a small scale example. Schmale and Iker tested the theory that hopelessness was a predictor of cervical cancer, using a directed interviewing technique and obtaining very positive results.[17] They also administered the Minnesota multiphasic personality inventory and the Rorschach inkblot test, with completely negative results. A miniscule meta-analysis of these three sets of data, treating them as if they had come from separate studies, would show a very small effect size of doubtful significance. Yet the interview was the only procedure relevant to the theory; the tests used are all purpose instruments of doubtful reliability and

69

validity. A hypothetico-deductive approach would say the study strongly supported the hypothesis when measures directed at the hypothesis were used to test it; both sets of test results are irrelevant (and would have been even if they had been positive).

This argument will be persuasive to anyone familiar with the critical literature concerning the Minnesota multiphasic personality inventory and the Rorschach test, yet how could a meta-analysis disregard these negative findings, other than by departing from its all inclusiveness and using what might look like subjective considerations? Undoubtedly, many investigators use multipurpose instruments like these tests to investigate specific hypotheses for which they are quite unsuited, and negative results so achieved are usually included in meta-analyses of data allegedly relevant to the original hypotheses.

*Adding apples and oranges*

Meta-analysis is only properly applicable if the data summarised are homogeneous—that is, treatment, patients, and end points must be similar or at least comparable. Yet often there is no evidence of any degree of such homogeneity and plenty of evidence to the contrary. Consider again the study by Smith *et al* concerned with "the benefits of psychotherapy."[6] Summarising over 500 papers, these authors came to the conclusion that "psychotherapy is beneficial, consistently so and in many different ways. Its benefits are on a par with other expensive and ambitious interventions, such as schooling and medicine . . . the evidence overwhelmingly supports the efficacy of psychotherapy . . . . Psychotherapy benefits people of all ages as reliably as schooling educates them, medicine cures them, or business turns a profit." Many reviews have repeated these statements with approbation, relying on the objectivity of meta-analysis. I have expressed a contrary view related to an earlier publication by the same authors, categorising it as "an exercise in mega-silliness."[9] Why such an unparliamentary expression?

In the studies analysed by Smith *et al* neither treatments, nor patients, nor end points were remotely comparable. Patients could be severe neurotics, mild neurotics, students suffering from a specific phobic anxiety, or people suffering from some form of existentialist discomfort. Treatments were exceedingly varied; indeed, a table gives 18 different types of treatment. End points were equally diverse, consisting of elimination of objective symptoms, psychiatric opinion, answers to a questionnaire, or some projective test like the Rorschach inkblot test.

Effect sizes summed over such exceedingly heterogeneous data can hardly be accorded any validity, yet these data are often cited as proving the efficacy of psychotherapy. A proper analysis would note that many different theories are involved in the way diverse treatments are used (psychodynamic, Adlerian, client centred, Gestalt, rational-emotive, transactional, reality therapy, behaviour therapy, etc) and would also note that if it is true, as the authors suggest, that all have won and all must have prizes (that is, that all do about equally well), then surely all the theories involved must be wrong. Each would predict that only methods of treatment based on the theory proposed would have positive results, or at least would surely outperform all the others; failure to do so constitutes disproof of the theory in question. And when we note that one of the alleged methods of treatment is "placebo therapy" then we must surely conclude that the success of placebo therapy, equal to that of psychodynamic, client centred, Adlerian, Gestalt, rational-emotive, and other therapies, suggests that all the effect of psychotherapy is due to placebo effects. (Actually the effects of behaviour therapy are significantly greater than the effects of the psychotherapies mentioned, and this has also emerged from a meta-analysis of German studies,[18] so there may be some positive results.) But the resolute search for some general effect for psychotherapy appears fruitless; the data used are too heterogeneous to be analysed.

## Inappropriate combining of studies

It is often the purpose of a meta-analysis to compare different causal factors (therapies, for example) in their effects. Thus Smith *et al*'s study compared behaviour therapy with different types of psychotherapy. In such a study all published accounts containing groups divided into no treatment and behaviour therapy, or no treatment and psychotherapy, would be compared. Doing so would pay no attention to the fact that different types of behaviour therapy are known to be appropriate for different types of symptoms. Thus desensitisation works with anxieties and phobias, while flooding with response prevention works well with obsessive-compulsive disorders; but vice versa, the results are quite disappointing.[19] Now consider a meta-analysis that would throw together studies that use the correct pairing with others that fail to do so. The resulting estimate of effect size would be strictly meaningless, averaging proper and improper uses of the method. Older studies were done before this difference in effectiveness became known; meta-analyses of (or including) older studies would come up with much lower estimates of the effect size than summaries of more recent studies. Experts would know things like that, but not all authors of meta-analyses are experts, and in any case textbooks on meta-analysis do not give guidance on how to incorporate such knowledge in the carrying out of the analysis.

## The theory directed approach

Concern with the truth or falsity of a given theory should make us look not at some measurement of effect size but rather at apparent anomalies and contradictions in the data, and at possible explanations of such contradictions. Consider some experiments reviewed elsewhere.[20] I had put forward a theory of introversion-extraversion which predicted that on a test of eyeblink conditioning introverts would perform much better than extraverts, and several experiments verified this prediction at a high level of significance. I also predicted that there would be no correlation with neuroticism-anxiety, and there was none. Very satisfactory.

At the same time Kenneth Spence, a well known psychologist at Iowa, predicted that neuroticism-anxiety would be related to quick and strong eyeblink conditioning, but introversion-extraversion would fail to show any relation to eyeblink conditioning. He too provided extensive evidence in favour of his theory. A typical meta-analysis would have shown very weak estimates of effect size for both our theories. Would that be a meaningful summary of the evidence? The obvious course to adopt would be to search for significant differences in the conduct of the experiment in an attempt to explain the observed differences in outcome (see chapter 5).

Nothing in the published accounts provided a suggestion, but when an independent observer visited both laboratories the answer became clear. In our work subjects were reassured, told that there would be no electric shocks; the apparatus that might frighten them was carefully hidden and every effort was made to eliminate anything that might cause anxiety. As a consequence, differences in anxiety proneness (neuroticism) had no chance to emerge, and hence the predicted effects of high cortical arousal in introverts were observed. Spence, on the other hand, failed to reassure his subjects, and in fact made every effort to exploit their proneness to anxiety. Consequently, high and low scorers on neuroticism showed very different degrees of anxiety, and these swamped any differential effects of cortical arousal. Clarifying discrepancies is more important than averaging estimates of effect size over discrepant data; however, such averaging is what occurs in typical meta-analyses.

## Summary

Newton wrote in a letter to Oldenburg in 1676: "For it is not number of Exp[ts], but weight to be regarded; where one will do, what need of many?" And Rutherford once pointed out that when you needed statistics to make your results significant, you would be better off doing a better experiment. Meta-analyses are often used to recover something from poorly designed studies, studies of insufficient statistical power, studies that give erratic results, and those resulting in apparent contradictions. Occasionally, meta-analysis does give worthwhile results, but all too often it is subject to methodological criticisms, some of which have been discussed above.

Careful workers can of course avoid these errors, but in doing so they will often violate the paradigms on which the whole notion of meta-analysis is built, and then will incur the accusation of subjectivity. Systematic reviews range all the way from highly subjective "traditional" methods to computer-like, completely objective counts of estimates of effect size over all published (and often unpublished) material regardless of quality. Neither extreme seems desirable. There cannot be one best method for fields of study so diverse as those for which meta-analysis has been used. If a medical treatment has an effect so recondite and obscure as to require meta-analysis to establish it, I would not be happy to have it used on me. It would seem better to improve the treatment, and the theory underlying the treatment.

1 Hedges LV, Olkin I. *Statistical methods for meta-analysis.* New York: Academic Press, 1985.
2 Huque MF. Experiences with meta-analysis in NDA submissions. *Proceedings of the Biopharmaceutical Section of the American Statistical Association* 1982; 2: 28–33.

3 Spitzer WO. Meta-analysis: unanswered questions about aggregating data. *J Clin Epidemiol* 1991; **44**: 103–7.

4 Slavin RE. Best-evidence synthesis: an alternative to meta-analysis and traditional reviews. *Educational Research* 1986; **15**: 9–11.

5 Eysenck HJ. Meta-analysis: an abuse of research integration. *Journal of Special Education* 1984; **18**: 41–59.

6 Smith ML, Glass GV, Miller TI. *The benefits of psychotherapy.* Baltimore: Johns Hopkins Press, 1980.

7 Knipschild P. Systematic reviews—some examples. *BMJ* 1994; **309**: 719–21. (Chapter 2)

8 Eysenck HJ. Meta-analysis: sense or non-sense? *Pharmaceutical Medicine* 1992; **6**: 113–19.

9 Eysenck HJ. An exercise in mega-silliness. *Am Psychol* 1978; **33**: 517.

10 Glass GV, Smith ML. Meta-analysis of research on class size and achievement. *Educational evolution and policy analysis* 1979; **1**: 2–16.

11 National Research Council. *Environmental tobacco smoke: measuring exposure and assessing health effects.* Washington: National Academy Press, 1986.

12 Fleiss JL, Gross AJ. Meta-analysis in epidemiology, with special reference to studies of the association between exposure to environmental tobacco smoke and lung cancer: a critique. *J Clin Epidemiol* 1991; **44**: 127, 439.

13 Stein RA. Meta-analysis from one FOA reviewer's perspective. *Proceedings of the biopharmaceutical section of the American Statistical Association* 1988; **2**: 34–8.

14 Janerich DT, Thompson WD, Varela LR, Greenwald P, Chorost S, Tucci C, et al. Lung cancer and exposure to tobacco smoke in the household. *N Engl J Med* 1990; **323**: 632–6.

15 Eysenck HJ. *Smoking, personality and stress: psychosocial factors in the prevention of cancer and coronary heart disease.* New York: Springer Verlag, 1991.

16 Lee PN. *Misclassification of smoking habits and passive smoking.* New York: Springer Verlag: 1988.

17 Schmale AH, Iker W. Hopelessness as a predictor of cervical cancer. *Soc Sci Med* 1971; **5**: 95–100.

18 Wittmann W, Matt G. Meta-analyse als Integration von Forschungsergebnissen am Beispiel deutschsprachiger Arbeiten zur Effektivität von Psychotherapie. *Psychologische Rundschau* 1986; **37**: 20–40.

19 Eysenck HJ, Martin I. *Theoretical foundations of behaviour therapy.* New York: Plenum Press, 1987.

20 Eysenck HJ, ed. *A model for personality.* New York: Springer Verlag, 1981.

# 7 Checklists for review articles

ANDREW D OXMAN

## Summary

Preparing a review entails many judgments. The focus of the review must be decided. Studies that are relevant to the focus of the review must be identified, selected for inclusion and critically appraised. Information must be collected and synthesised from the relevant studies, and conclusions must be drawn. Checklists can help prevent important errors in this process. Reviewers, editors, content experts, and users of reviews all have a role to play in improving the quality of published reviews and promoting the appropriate use of reviews by decisionmakers. It is essential that both providers and users appraise the validity of review articles.

## Why checklists?

When we think about flying, it is obvious why a checklist is used before take off. Airplanes are complex machines. Things can go wrong with them, and it is preferable that problems are discovered on the ground. However brilliant a pilot and crew might be, most of us would prefer that they use a checklist when preparing for take off, rather than relying on memory.

The need for checklists for review articles is less obvious, but the rationale is much the same. Preparing a review is a complex process entailing many judgments. The focus of the review must be decided. Studies that are relevant to the focus of the review must be identified, selected for inclusion, and critically appraised.

75

Information must be collected and synthesised from the relevant studies, and conclusions must be drawn. Many decisions must be made throughout this process.

It is important to go through this process systematically to avoid errors. Explicitness about how decisions were made enables others to assess how well the process protected against errors. Checklists can help those doing and using reviews to avoid important errors.

Faulty reviews may not seem as perilous as faulty airplanes. However, if people are going to use reviews to guide decisions about health care, misleading reviews can indeed be deadly. On the other hand, if people are not going to use reviews to guide decisions, why bother with them?

Before deciding that we should not bother with reviews, it is important to remember that there is little choice. Whether we rely on published, formal reviews or reviews done inside our heads, or the heads of experts, the risks remain. The same judgments must be made, whether explicitly or implicitly. The advantage of using carefully done, systematic reviews becomes clear when we observe how often mistakes are made when research is reviewed non-systematically, whether by experts or others. The costs of mistaken conclusions based on non-systematic reviews can be high.

Life saving treatments, such as thrombolytic therapy and aspirin for patients with myocardial infarctions, can go unused. Other treatments that do not have proved benefits and may even be harmful, such as calcium channel blockers and antiarrhythmic agents for patients with myocardial infarctions, can be used inappropriately.[1]

## What should be checked?

The most dangerous errors in reviews are systematic ones (bias) rather than ones that occur by chance alone (random errors). Consequently, the most important thing for doers and users of a review to check is its "validity": the extent to which its design and conduct are likely to have protected against bias.

Random errors can also be deadly. However, if a review is done systematically and quantitative results are presented, the confidence interval around the results provides a good indication of "precision": the extent to which the results are likely to differ from the "truth" because of chance alone.[2] A confidence interval does not provide any indication of the likelihood of bias.

Other attributes of a review are also important, including choice of focus, degree of innovation in the approach, potential impact on future scientific developments, literary quality, and handling of pertinent ethical issues. It may or may not be appropriate to include items related to these attributes in a checklist. This depends on the purpose of the particular checklist.

*Asking the questions*

For most, if not all purposes, the first question that should be addressed by a checklist is, is the focus of this review relevant? This question can only be answered relative to a specific context— for example, whether it is relevant to a particular patient, practice setting, or readership. The next question should be, are the results likely to be valid? If there are important concerns about validity, any other considerations are largely irrelevant.

A number of "checklists" have been published suggesting what should be examined when assessing the validity of a review.[3-10] There are some differences in the items included in these lists and in how each item is addressed, but they all focus on the same sources of bias (box 1): how the problem was formulated; how studies were identified, selected for inclusion, and critically appraised; how data were collected and synthesised; and how the results were interpreted. Some questions relating to each potential source of bias are listed in box 1.

Several authors have examined issues pertaining to the validity of reviews,[5-13] and many of these issues are considered in the other articles in this series. The logic behind the questions in the box, and other questions that can be asked about how well a review has protected against bias, is straightforward. Preparing a review of research is in itself a research process. It is a type of survey, and the scientific principles underlying reviews and epidemiological surveys are the same. In a review a question must be posed, a target population of information sources identified and accessed, appropriate information obtained from that population in an unbiased fashion, and conclusions derived. Often statistical analysis (meta-analysis) can help in reaching conclusions.

The starting point for any research project is to ask a good question and develop a protocol laying out the methods that will

## Box 1—Sources of bias and methods of protecting against bias

Problem formulation
- Is the question clearly focused?

Study identification
- Is the search for relevant studies thorough?

Study selection
- Are the inclusion criteria appropriate?

Appraisal of studies
- Is the validity of included studies adequately assessed?

Data collection
- Is missing information obtained from investigators?

Data synthesis
- How sensitive are the results to changes in the way the review is done?

Interpretation of results
- Do the conclusions flow from the evidence that is reviewed?

- Are recommendations linked to the strength of the evidence?

- Are judgments about preferences (values) explicit?

- If there is "no evidence of effect" is caution taken not to interpret this as "evidence of no effect"?

- Are subgroup analyses interpreted cautiously?

be used to address the question. Without a clearly focused question there is little point in going further. The types of people, interventions, and outcomes of interest should all be clearly specified.

*Including studies*

The criteria used to select studies for inclusion in a review should be consistent with the focus. They should be explicit to protect against biased selection of studies. Similarly, the criteria that are used to assess the validity of the studies that are included should be explicit to minimise biased assessments and weighting of the included studies.

Variation in quality can explain variation in the results of the included studies. Statistical summaries (meta-analyses) of results from studies of variable quality can result in a "false positive" conclusion (concluding that there is an effect when in truth there is not) if the less rigorous studies that are included are biased towards overestimating the effectiveness of the intervention being evaluated. Such summaries might also result in a "false negative" conclusion (concluding that there is not an effect when in truth there is) if the less rigorous studies provide less precise or biased estimates of the effects of the intervention, thereby obscuring the true effect.[14] The methodological quality of the included studies is important even if the results or quality of the included studies do not vary. If the evidence is consistent but all the studies are flawed, the conclusions of the review would not be nearly as strong as if consistent results were obtained from a series of high quality studies.

Poor quality studies and insufficient reporting are, unfortunately, common in the medical literature.[15-20] Information obtained through personal communication can strengthen the results of a review. To avoid introducing bias, unpublished information that is obtained should be unambiguous; it should be obtained in writing and coded in the same fashion as published information.

*Analysing the data*

The analysis or synthesis of the data that are collected for a systematic review entails the whole process of evaluating and synthesising the results of the included studies. Statistical techniques may or may not be used. The statistical techniques used in meta-analyses do not differ in principle from those used in primary research,[21] and the logic behind their use is the same. Statistical analysis is a tool which, when used appropriately, can help us to derive meaningful conclusions from data and to avoid analytic errors. Like any tool, it can also be misused.

Because there are different approaches to conducting a systematic review, it is important to ask how sensitive the results are to changes in the way the review is done. Such "sensitivity analyses" provide an approach to testing how robust the results of a review are relative to key decisions and assumptions that were made in the process of conducting the review. The types of decisions and assumptions that might be examined in sensitivity analyses include:

- Changing the inclusion criteria
- Including or excluding trials where there is some ambiguity as to whether they meet the inclusion criteria
- Excluding unpublished studies
- Excluding studies of lower methodological quality
- Reanalysing the data by using a reasonable range of results for trials in which there may be some uncertainty about the results
- Reanalysing the data imputing a reasonable range of values for missing data
- Reanalysing the data using different statistical approaches.

Even when the results of a review are robust, it is possible to reach erroneous conclusions if the results are misinterpreted. The last five questions in the table all focus on this source of bias. They need little elaboration but deserve close attention.

*Conclusions and recommendations*

The conclusions of a review should not exceed the evidence that is reviewed. So far as possible, recommendations should be linked to the strength of the evidence. Preferably, this should be done with an explicit approach to specify levels of evidence—for example, like the one used by the Antithrombotic Therapy Consensus Conference (box 2).[22]

---

## Box 2—Levels of evidence for treatment

Level I  The lower limit of the confidence interval for the effect of treatment from a systematic review of randomised controlled trials exceeded the clinically significant benefit.

Level II  The lower limit of the confidence interval for the effect of treatment from a systematic review of randomised controlled trials fell below the clinically significant benefit (but the point estimate of its effect was at or above the clinically significant benefit)

Level III  Non-randomised concurrent cohort studies

Level IV  Non-randomised historical cohort studies

Level V  Case series

Detailed definitions for these levels of evidence and corresponding grades of recommendations are provided by Cook *et al*[22]

---

Because health care interventions entail costs and risks of harm as well as expectations of benefit, practice recommendations require judgments about preferences (the values attached to different outcomes) in addition to judgments about evidence.[23] When conclusions involve judgments about preferences this should be clearly stated. For example, women considering hormone replacement therapy must consider the tradeoffs between the potential benefits (prevention of hip fracture and cardiovascular disease) and the possible harm (breast and endometrial cancer and vaginal bleeding).[24] [25] The relative value attached to these outcomes varies from woman to woman. Before drawing conclusions for clinical practice, a systematic review of the effects of preventive hormone therapy must consider all of the potentially important outcomes. Assumptions about the relative value of these should not be hidden.

### Errors

The last two questions in box 1 refer to two common types of error that are found in reviews (and elsewhere). One is to confuse "no evidence of effect" with "evidence of no effect." For example, no evidence that love causes heartbreak is not the same as evidence that love causes no heartbreak.

The other type of error is misinterpretation of subgroup analyses. It is frequently of interest in a review to examine a particular category of participants—for example, women, a certain age group, or those with a specific pattern of disease. These examinations, or subgroup analyses, are exceedingly common, but they are also often misleading.[26] [27] Conclusions based on subgroup analyses can do harm both when a particular category of people is denied effective treatment (a false negative conclusion), and when ineffective or even harmful treatment is given to a subgroup of people (a false positive conclusion). Subgroup analyses can also generate misleading recommendations about directions for future research that, if they are followed, can waste scarce resources. Because of these risks and the frequency of their occurrence, it is important to be cautious when enticed to perform and interpret subgroup analyses.

## Who should check?

Traditionally, reviews have been written by experts on the topic (content experts). When seeking critiques of review articles (peer review), editors have looked to other content experts in the field for help. These policies may seem intuitively reasonable and appropriate. However, there are reasons for serious scepticism. Content experts may lack the objectivity desirable in preparing or critiquing a review article. For example, personal experience in primary research is highly salient and considerably more vivid than the research of others, and therefore likely to be given undue weight in judgments.[28] This is also true for personal clinical experience.

In examining the relation of content expertise to the quality of review articles, Guyatt and I found that content expertise in an area was inversely related to methodological quality: the greater the content expertise of the author, the poorer the quality of the review.[29] This might have been related to the strength of prior opinions and the amount of time spent preparing a review article. Content experts tended to have stronger opinions about the topic of a review and to spend less time preparing a review.

We also found poor agreement about the methodological quality of reviews among content experts.[29] At least two explanations for this are possible: lack of training, or the effects of expertise. In either case, the results cast doubt on the wisdom of relying exclusively on content experts in a clinical area who do not have specific methodological training to check the quality of reviews.

Mulrow, in her classic study of the quality of review articles in the medical literature, has shown the failure of traditional review articles to describe their methods.[6] Of even greater concern, Antman and colleagues in another enlightening study showed the extent to which the conclusions of content experts can differ from those based on the results of systematic reviews.[1] An extreme interpretation of findings such as these might be that content experts should occupy themselves with the task of producing new data or else retire from the topics of their expertise[30] and leave the task of preparing and critiquing review articles to those who have specific training in the science of research reviews. A more reasonable interpretation might be to acknowledge the importance of content expertise while at the same time recognising the need for others to play a role in ensuring the quality of reviews.

### Roles for content experts

Content experts often belong to an "invisible college" of people who interact with each other because of a common interest in an

Table 7.1 *Who should check what?*

| | Reviewers | Editors | Content experts | Users |
|---|---|---|---|---|
| Focus | ✓ | ✓ | | ✓ |
| Missing studies | ✓ | ✓ | ✓ | |
| Selection criteria | ✓ | ✓ | | ✓ |
| Quality of studies | ✓ | ✓ | | |
| Data collection | ✓ | ✓ | | |
| Synthesis of data | ✓ | ✓ | | |
| Interpretation | ✓ | ✓ | ✓ | ✓ |

area of research. Because of these connections, content experts may be aware of studies that reviewers might otherwise miss. Content experts often have extensive knowledge of related evidence outside the specific focus of a review and practical experience in their area of expertise. They may be more aware of nuances than others. Hence they can bring important perspectives to the interpretation of the results of a review.

In summary, content experts have an important role in ensuring the quality of reviews, but we cannot rely on their expertise alone (table 7.1). Reviewers and editors, especially, must check whether the methods used in a review are likely to protect against bias. This is essential if the quality of published review articles is to improve. In addition, users of reviews must be able to judge whether a review is clearly focused—and whether that focus is relevant to their situation. They must be able to judge whether the studies included in a review are appropriately selected relative to the focus. Finally, they must be able to ensure that the conclusions that are drawn on the basis of a review, whether the reviewers' or their own, are supported by the evidence that is reviewed.

To take well informed decisions about health care, people at all levels of the health service need access to systematic reviews of the relevant evidence. Reviewers, editors, content experts, and users of reviews all need to check that review articles are valid if we want to make decisions based on evidence rather than on authority.[31-33]

The author received support for this work from the Nuffield Provincial Hospitals Trust as a UK Cochrane Centre Visiting Fellow.

1 Antman EM, Lau J, Kupelnick B, Mosteller F, Chalmers TC. A comparison of results of meta-analyses of randomized control trials and recommendations of clinical experts: treatments for myocardial evaluation. *JAMA* 1992; **268**: 240–8.

2 Altman DG. Confidence intervals in research evaluation. *Ann Intern Med* 1992; **116** (suppl 2): A28.

3 Jackson GB. Methods for integrative reviews. *Review of Education Research* 1980; **50**: 438–60.

4 Cooper H. Scientific guidelines for conducting integrative research reviews. *Review of Education Research* 1982; **52**: 291–302.

5 Light RJ, Pillemer DB. *Summing up: the science of reviewing research.* Cambridge, MA: Harvard University Press, 1984: 160–73.

6 Mulrow CD. The medical review article: state of the science. *Ann Intern Med* 1987; **106**: 485–8.

7 Sacks HS, Berrier J, Reitman D, Ancona-Berk VA, Chalmers TC, et al . Meta-analyses of randomized controlled trials. *N Engl J Med* 1987; **316**: 450–5.

8 L'Abbé KA, Detsky AS, O'Rourke K. Meta-analysis in clinical research. *Ann Intern Med* 1987; **107**: 224–33.

9 Oxman AD, Guyatt GH. Guidelines for reading literature reviews. *Can Med Assoc J* 1988; **138**: 697–703.

10 Oxman AD, Cooke DJ, Guyatt GH. Users' guides to the medical literature. VI. How to use an overview. *JAMA* 1994; **272**: 1367–71.

11 Glass GV, McGaw B, Smith M. *Meta-analysis in social research.* Newbury Park: Sage, 1981.

12 Yusuf S, Simon R, Ellenberg S, eds. Proceedings of "Methodologic Issues in Overviews of Randomized Clinical Trials." *Stat Med* 1987; **6**: 217–409.

13 Cooper H, Hedges LV, eds. *The handbook of research synthesis.* New York: Russell Sage Foundation, 1993.

14 Detsky AS, Naylor CD, O'Rourke K, McGee AJ, L'Abbé KA. Incorporating variations in the quality of individual randomized trials into meta-analysis. *J Clin Epidemiol* 1992; **45**: 255–65.

15 Williamson JW, Goldschmidt PG, Colton T. The quality of medical literature: an analysis of validation assessments. In: Bailar JC, Mosteller F, eds. *Medical uses of statistics.* Waltham, MA: NEJM Books, 1986: 370–91.

16 Fletcher RH, Fletcher SW. Clinical research in general medical journals: a 30 year perspective. *N Engl J Med* 1979; **301**: 180–3.

17 Mosteller F, Gilbert JP, McPeek B. Reporting standards and research strategies for controlled trials: agenda for the editor. *Controlled Clin Trials* 1980; **1**: 37–57.

18 Gøtzsche PC. Methodology and overt and hidden bias in reports on 196 double-blind trials of nonsteroidal antiinflammatory drugs in rheumatoid arthritis. *Controlled Clin Trials* 1989; **10**: 31–56.

19 Emerson JD, Burdick E, Hoaglin DC, Mosteller F, Chalmers TC. An empirical study of the possible relation of treatment differences to quality scores in controlled randomized clinical trials. *Controlled Clin Trials* 1990; **11**: 339–52.

20 Schulz KF, Chalmers I, Hayes RJ, Altman DG. Empirical evidence of bias: dimensions of methodological quality are associated with estimates of treatment effects. *JAMA* 1995; **273**: 408–12.

21 Laird NM, Mosteller F. Some statistical methods for combining experimental results. *Int J Technology Assess Health Care* 1990; **6**: 5–30.

22 Cook DJ, Guyatt GH, Laupacis A, Sackett DL. Rules of evidence and clinical recommendations on the use of antithrombotic agents. Antithrombotic Therapy Consensus Conference. *Chest* 1992; **102**: 305–11S.

23 Eddy DM. Anatomy of a decision. *JAMA* 1990; **263**: 441–3.

24 Grady D, Rubin SM, Petitti DB, Fox CS, Black D, Ettinger B, et al. Hormone therapy to prevent disease and prolong life in postmenopausal women. *Ann Intern Med* 1992; **117**: 1016–37.

25 American College of Physicians. Guidelines for counselling postmenopausal women about preventive hormone therapy. *Ann Intern Med* 1992; **117**: 1038–41.

26 Yusuf S, Wittes J, Probstfield J, Tyroler HA. Analysis and interpretation of treatment effects in subgroups of patients in randomized clinical trials. *JAMA* 1991; **266**: 93–8.

27 Oxman AD, Guyatt GH. A consumer's guide to subgroup analyses. *Ann Intern Med* 1992; **116**: 78–84.

28 Cooper HM. On the social psychology of using research review: the case of desegregation and the black achiever. In: Feldman RS, ed. *Social psychology of education.* Cambridge: Cambridge University Press, 1986; **341**: 341–63.

29 Oxman AD, Güyatt GH. The science of reviewing research. *Ann NY Acad Sci* 1993; **703**: 125–31.
30 Sackett DL. Proposals for the health sciences. I. Compulsory retirement for experts. *J Chron Dis* 1983; **36**: 545–7.
31 Evidence-based Medicine Working Group. Evidence-based medicine: a new approach to teaching the practice of medicine. *JAMA* 1992; **268**: 2420–5.
32 Guyatt GH, Rennie D. Users' guides to the medical literature. *JAMA* 1993; **270**: 2096–7.
33 Oxman AD, Sackett DL, Guyatt GH. Users' guides to the medical literature. I. How to get started. *JAMA* 1993; **270**: 2093–5.

# 8 Reporting, updating, and correcting systematic reviews of the effects of health care

IAIN CHALMERS, BRIAN HAYNES

## Summary

The recent growth in the numbers of published systematic reviews reflects growing recognition of their importance for improving knowledge about the effects of health care. The Cochrane Collaboration—an international network of individuals and institutions—has evolved to prepare systematic, periodically updated reviews of randomised controlled trials and of observational evidence when this is appropriate. The large amount of existing evidence that needs to be considered creates a problem for the reporting of systematic reviews: the need to ensure that methods and results of systematic reviews are adequately described has to be reconciled with the limited space available in printed journals. A possible solution is the use of electronic publications: reviews can be published simultaneously in a short, printed form and in a more detailed electronic form. Electronic publications also have the advantage that reviews can be updated as new evidence becomes available or mistakes are identified.

86

# Primary and secondary research on the effects of health care: the dangerous consequences of double standards

It was not until very recently that anyone drew attention to the fact that clinical investigators usually jettison scientific principles when they move from primary research to secondary research (reviews). Mulrow, in 1987, first showed that this double standard was manifest in some of the world's leading medical journals,[1] and Huth, in an accompanying editorial in *Annals of Internal Medicine*, said that something ought to be done about it.[2] The following year Oxman and Guyatt published guidelines to help people to judge the scientific quality and trustworthiness of reviews.[3]

The failure of clinical investigators to apply scientific principles to control biases and imprecision in their reviews of evidence about the effects of care can have serious consequences. For example, in 1987 the second edition of the *Oxford Textbook of Medicine* advised its tens of thousands of readers that "The clinical benefits of thrombolysis [in treating patients with myocardial infarction] whether expressed as improved patient survival or preservation of left ventricular function, remain to be established."[4] This unsupported view appeared four years after Yusuf and his colleagues had shown in a systematic review of the relevant randomised controlled trials that this treatment reduced the risk of premature death after myocardial infaction,[5][6] Indeed, as was shown subsequently by Antman and his colleagues, strong evidence in support of thrombolysis would have emerged a decade earlier had a systematic review been conducted then.[7]

This is just one of many examples that could be used to illustrate the importance of systematic and timely reviews of evidence about the effects of health care. When the research community synthesises existing evidence thoroughly, it is certain that a substantial proportion of current notions about the effects of health care will be changed. Forms of care currently believed to be ineffective will be shown to be effective; forms of care thought to be useful will be exposed as either useless or harmful; and the justification for uncertainty about the effects of many other forms of care will be made explicit. In addition, systematic reviews of existing evidence will reveal that many proposals for new research are misguided because they have not taken proper account of available information.

Systematic reviews of existing evidence, using meta-analysis when appropriate and possible, are examples of "advanced clinical research."[8] Because reviews have such an important place in the chain linking basic research and improved human health, the science of reviewing research must be recognised more explicitly, both within the academic community and more widely.

There is encouraging evidence that this proposition is beginning to be accepted in several places. Using the term meta-analysis as a marker for tracking growth in interest in systematic methods of review, a Medline search before 1982 could be expected to yield about one systematic review a year. Between 1982 and 1985 the average annual yield was about 15.[9] Since 1986, however, the number has increased dramatically, and a Medline search using the MeSH term META-ANALYSIS and the text word "meta-analysis" yielded over 500 citations published in 1992 (C Lefebvre, personal communication). The National Library of Medicine acknowledged this advance in 1993 when the term was given the status of a publication type.

This growth in the numbers of systematic reviews certainly reflects both growing recognition of their importance within academia and support from the organisations that employ clinical investigators. Support for systematic reviews has come, in addition, from those who are trying to assemble information that will help to make more effective use of limited resources for health care. For example, in the United States, the Agency for Health Care Policy and Research—part of the Public Health Service—has invested substantially in reviews of existing evidence about the effects of care, and in the United Kingdom, the NHS R&D programme has established two centres (in Oxford and York) to help to prepare systematic reviews of existing information. At an international level, a network of individuals and institutions—the Cochrane Collaboration—has evolved in response to Cochrane's criticism of the health professions for not having organised systematic, periodically updated reviews of all relevant randomised controlled trials.[10]

*Cochrane reviews*

Publication of Cochrane reviews in pilot form began in 1993 with the release of a specialised database[11] compiled using subsets of reviews contained in the "parent" *Cochrane Database of Systematic Reviews*. Publication of the *Cochrane Database of*

*Systematic Reviews* itself, although initially containing only a small number of reviews covering a relatively narrow range of topics, began in 1995.

The magnitude of the task of finding out what can be known from existing evidence about the effects of health care should not be underestimated: it seems likely that, even if attention were to be focused on randomised controlled trials alone, as many as a million studies conducted during the second half of the 20th century may need to be considered. Hundreds of people are already contributing to the Cochrane Collaboration and getting to grips with Archie Cochrane's daunting agenda; but it is likely that it will take at least a couple of decades for a stable state to be reached such that the results of new primary research are being incorporated efficiently into an existing body of systematic reviews of previous research.

At least one commentator has pointed out that a case could be made for a moratorium on proposals for additional primary research until existing results of research have been incorporated in scientifically defensible reviews.[12] This view is reflected in the fact that some funding bodies have begun to make it clear to potential applicants that they will expect applications for support for new research to be accompanied by systematic reviews of relevant existing evidence. These sytematic reviews must show that the proposed new research is necessary and that it has been designed appropriately—in brief, that it is likely to constitute a sensible use of the limited resources available for research.

## Reporting systematic reviews of the effects of health care

Many journal editors are responding to suggestions about how they can serve the needs of their readers more effectively,[13] [14] and one of the ways that they are doing so is by accepting the need to improve the scientific quality of the reviews that they publish.[2] This trend has had consequences for reports of primary research as well as for "stand alone" reviews because there is an increasing expectation among readers that investigators will set the results of new primary research in the context of systematic reviews of relevant existing evidence.

This trend has meant that reports of reviews, whether they

stand alone or are components of the discussion sections of reports of new primary research, now tend to take up more space than previously. When the totality of relevant evidence requiring review is small, this does not present any great problems.[15] When, as is increasingly the case, there is a large amount of existing evidence, journal editors are confronted with a dilemma. On the one hand, they need to ensure that the materials, methods, and results of systematic reviews are reported in sufficient detail to allow readers to assess their scientific quality; on the other hand, these scientific requirements have to be reconciled with constraints imposed by the inevitably limited space available in printed journals. The 29 page, two part *Lancet* report of the Early Breast Cancer Trialists' Collaborative Group, and the 46 page, three part *BMJ* report of the Antiplatelet Trialists' Collaboration, are recent examples of the opportunities and problems confronting editors.[16 17]

The editorial dilemma was made explicit soon after the dawn of the new era of systematic reviews of randomised controlled trials. The 10 page report in the *Lancet* of the ISIS-1 trial included a discussion section incorporating a systematic review of all the trials of $\beta$ blockade for myocardial infarction.[18] This provided an up to date assessment of the available evidence and showed how the results of the new trial contributed to the overall picture. While acknowledging that there was a good case for presenting such analyses in the discussion sections of reports of primary research, an accompanying editorial warned that the *Lancet* would lead the opposition to anyone suggesting that such "lengthy tailpieces" should become a regular feature of clinical trial reports.[19]

*Electronic opportunities*

As it happens, it has been the *Lancet* (among the major general medical journals) that has been most active in exploring how best to resolve these dilemmas. The *Lancet* published correspondence in response to its 1986 editorial and subsequently which drew attention to the potential for exploiting simultaneous electronic and paper publication of lengthy systematic reviews.[20 21] Within a month of the launch of the first electronically published general medical journal—the *Online Journal of Current Clinical Trials*—in 1992, the *Lancet* announced that it had come to an arrangement with the new journal whereby certain reports, including systematic reviews of trials, would be published simultaneously both in short, printed forms and in more detailed electronic forms.[22] The first examples of this arrangement for parallel publication of detailed and brief reports of systematic reviews were published the following year.[23][24]

The principle of concurrent electronic and paper publication of systematic reviews has been reflected in the arrangements agreed by the Cochrane Collaboration with the *BMJ* and the *Lancet*, and subsequently with other journals, such as *Annals of Internal Medicine*. The International Committee of Medical Journal Editors (the Vancouver Group) has also supported the arrangement. The detailed, highly structured reports of systematic reviews prepared for dissemination electronically in the *Cochrane Database of Systematic Reviews* are eligible for submission to any print journals endorsing these arrangements. If, after assessment, a print journal accepts a Cochrane review for publication, it will be shortened and modified to reflect the style and other requirements of the journal concerned. This shortened and modified version of the review will then be published concurrently with the electronic dissemination of a longer, more structured version through the *Cochrane Database of Systematic Reviews*.

Full success in reporting the findings of systematic reviews will not be achieved by these means alone.[25][26] Improvements are needed in the integration of information from reviews in the development and reporting of clinical guidelines and health policy. There is also a need for innovation in reporting of review findings in medical textbooks, in materials for the continuing education of health professionals, patients, and the public, and in computerised clinical decision support systems.[27] Some of these innovations have already been piloted in the preparation of a popular guide to the detailed Cochrane reviews of care in pregnancy and childbirth,[28] and in the development of clinical and policy guidelines based on them. As the number and variety of systematic reviews grows there will be an increasing need for refined indexing to permit easy retrieval and for organising the reviews in ways that allow them to be easily rearranged to meet particular needs.

## Updating and correcting systematic reviews of the effects of health care

A combination of electronic and paper publication will help

people to cope with the sheer size of many reports of systematic reviews. Electronic media come into their own, however, when systematic reviews must be updated or corrected as new evidence becomes available and mistakes are identified.[19] It is often frustrating for authors (and others) that the printed reports of their reviews cannot be amended when omissions and mistakes are discovered and drawn to their attention. Because these printed reports will often be reproduced in offprints and photocopies and bound in books and library collections, it is inevitable that many readers will be misled, often over a period of many years. Diligent readers wishing to be properly informed must assemble the original reports, together with the correction notices, letters to the editor, and other criticisms and responses published subsequently, and then try to prepare an effective synthesis of all this material. These are difficult and tedious tasks, particularly when the criticisms and comments are widely scattered.

It is essential that more efficient arrangements are developed for criticising and amending reviews in the light of new evidence and valid criticisms. To achieve this, the Cochrane Collaboration's working methods include a commitment to timely updating and concurrent reporting of criticisms and other responses. This commitment is backed up by the cover sheet for each review contained in the *Cochrane Database of Systematic Reviews*, which gives the names, addresses, and other contact details (telephone, fax, and electronic mail) both of the principal reviewer and of the editorial team responsible for coordinating the collaborative review group to which he or she belongs.

These requirements of those contributing to the Cochrane Collaboration, taken together with the practical experience acquired by a group of reviewers preparing and maintaining systematic reviews of controlled trials in pregnancy and childbirth,[29 30] lie behind the Cochrane Collaboration's adoption of electronic media as a primary means of assembling and disseminating Cochrane reviews.[31] As it evolves, the Collaboration intends to create an iterative system through which successive versions of each review will reflect not only the emergence of new data but also valid criticisms, solicited or unsolicited, from whatever source.[30]

*An interactive system*

The use of successive issues on floppy disk and CD-ROM to

update and amend Cochrane reviews in the light of new evidence and criticisms undoubtedly represents an advance beyond the constraints imposed by publishing reviews in print. It will be important to go beyond these arrangements, however, to develop more efficient and transparent mechanisms for maximising the reliability of Cochrane reviews. Efficient online access to the *Cochrane Database of Systematic Reviews* would seem to provide the most satisfactory basis for this. It should be possible for people consulting the database to append their criticisms and comments to the Cochrane reviews, for the attention not only of Cochrane reviewers and editors but also the readers of the reviews. Although those consulting the Cochrane database would be offered the most recent version of a review as the default option, earlier versions of each review, together with any intervening criticisms, would be archived electronically for consultation if desired. Complementary arrangements will be needed to ensure that other publication forms that use Cochrane reviews are aware of substantive updates.

Although an interactive system of the kind outlined above may take some years to develop, the scientific dividends could be substantial. It should facilitate the critical dialogues on which advances in knowledge so often depend. There is certainly no room for complacency about the existing arrangements for critical assessment of material submitted to and published in scientific journals.[32] Electronic publishing can be exploited to extend this critical assessment beyond the handful of individuals selected by journal editors as referees before publication and the handful of correspondents offered space in correspondence columns after publication.

## Prospects and challenges

Systematic reviews of research evidence will play an increasing role in the evolution of health services, the design and justification of controlled trials in health care, and the education of health professionals and lay people. The Cochrane Collaboration is helping to promote the development of systematic reviews by setting explicit standards for reviews; by providing a framework within which people can collaborate in preparing and maintaining reviews in areas of mutual interest; by helping to mobilise resources of various kinds for reviewers; and by developing better means for disseminating systematic reviews to all those who may find them helpful. Medical journals and publishers are playing their part through featuring systematic reviews and by fostering favourable copyright arrangements.

Substantial challenges remain, however. Relatively few health care problems have been covered by systematic reviews so far, and access to existing reviews is limited. The demand for systematic reviews vastly exceeds the capacity of those who are prepared to commit themselves not only to preparing reviews which meet acceptable scientific standards but to the long term maintenance of these reviews as new evidence and criticisms emerge. Funding agencies and academic institutions are only just beginning to treat systematic reviews as scientific projects in their own right: for comparable effort, the current rewards for people engaged in primary research remain significantly better than those for people preparing systematic reviews. Traditional textbooks based on opinion and unsystematic reviews continue to be published in vast numbers.

These problems will be overcome as the value of systematic reviews becomes more widely known and as the infrastructure for development, organisation, and dissemination of reviews becomes better established. It will take a concerted effort over many years to reach the point at which existing evidence about the effects of health care has been organised systematically and made readily available to the variety of people who need this information to help them take better decisions in health care and research, but there is every reason to believe that the effort required will be seen to have been worthwhile.

Iain Chalmers is supported by the NHS R&D Programme; Brian Haynes is supported by the Canadian National Research and Development Programme and McMaster University. The Cochrane Collaboration is an international network of individuals and institutions receiving support from a wide variety of sources. The steering group of the Cochrane Collaboration is chaired by Professor David Sackett, formerly at McMaster University, Canada, now at the Nuffield Department of Medicine, University of Oxford.

1 Mulrow CD. The medical review article: state of the science. *Ann Intern Med* 1987; **104:** 485–8.
2 Huth EJ. Needed: review articles with more scientific rigor. *Ann Intern Med* 1987; **106:** 470–1.
3 Oxman AD, Guyatt GH. Guidelines for reading literature reviews. *Can Med Assoc J* 1988; **138:** 697–703.
4 Pentecost BL. Myocardial infarction. In: Weatherall DJ, Ledingham JGG, Warrell DA,

eds. *Oxford textbook of medicine*. Vol 2. 2nd ed. Oxford: Oxford University Press, 1987: 13–173.

5 Yusuf S, Sleight P. Limitation of myocardial infarct size. *Drugs* 1983; **25**: 441–50.

6 Yusuf S, Collins R, Peto R, Furberg C, Stampfer MJ, Goldhaber SZ, *et al*. Intravenous and intracoronary fibrinolytic therapy in acute myocardial infarction. Overview of results on mortality, reinfarction and side effect from 33 randomized controlled trials. *Eur Heart J* 1985; **6**: 556–85.

7 Antman EM, Lau J, Kupelnick B, Mosteller F, Chalmers TC. A comparison of results of meta-analyses of randomized control trials and recommendations of clinical experts. *JAMA* 1992; **268**: 240–8.

8 Haynes RB. Loose connections between peer-reviewed clinical journals and clinical practice. *Ann Intern Med* 1990; **113**: 724–8.

9 Dickersin K, Higgins K, Meinert CL. Identification of meta-analyses: the need for standard terminology. *Controlled Clin Trials* 1990; **11**: 52–66.

10 Cochrane AL. 1931–1971: a critical review, with particular reference to the medical profession. In: Teeling-Smith G, ed. *Medicines for the year 2000*. London: Office of Health Economics, 1979: 1–11.

11 Cochrane Pregnancy and Childbirth Database [derived from *The Cochrane Database of Systematic Reviews;* published through Cochrane Updates on Disk]. Oxford: Update Software, 1993: Disk Issue 1.

12 Bausell BB. After the meta-analytic revolution. *Evaluation and the Health Professions* 1993; **16**: 3–12.

13 Smith R. What's wrong with the BMJ? [editor's choice]. *BMJ* 1994 January 8, **308**: i.

14 Haynes RB. How clinical journals could serve clinician readers better. In: Lock S, ed. *The future of medical journals*, London: BMJ, 1991: 116–26.

15 Saunders MC, Dick JS, Brown IMcL, McPherson K, Chalmers I. The effects of hospital admission for bed rest on the duration of twin pregnancy: a randomised trial. *Lancet* 1985; **ii**: 793–5.

16 Early Breast Cancer Trialists' Collaborative Group. Systemic treatment of early breast cancer by hormonal, cytotoxic, or immune therapy. *Lancet* 1992; **339**: 1–15, 71–85.

17 Antiplatelet Trialists' Collaboration. Secondary prevention of vascular disease by prolonged anti-platelet treatment. *BMJ* 1994; **308**: 81–107, 159–68, 235–46.

18 ISIS-1 Collaborative Group. Randomised trial of intravenous atenolol among 16,027 cases of suspected acute myocardial infarction: ISIS-1. *Lancet* 1986; **ii**: 57–66.

19 Intravenous beta-blockade during acute myocardial infarction [editorial]. *Lancet* 1986; **ii**: 79–80.

20 Chalmers I. Electronic publications for updating controlled trial reviews. *Lancet* 1986; **ii**: 287.

21 Lock S. Long reports. *Lancet* 1992; **339**: 249.

22 More brevity in The Lancet [editorial]. *Lancet* 1992; **340**: 519.

23 Wang PH, Lau J, Chalmers TC. Meta-analysis of effects of intensive blood-glucose control on late complications of type 1 diabetes. *Lancet* 1993; **341**: 1306–9.

24 Wang PH, Lau J, Chalmers TC. Meta-analysis of effects of intensive glycemic control on late complications of type 1 diabetes mellitus. *Online J Curr Clin Trials*, 1993 May 21: document No 60.

25 Lomas J, Sisk JE, Stocking B. From evidence to practice in the United States, the United Kingdom, and Canada. *Milbank Q* 1993; **71**: 405–10.

26 Patterson-Brown S, Wyatt JC, Fisk NM. Are clinicians interested in up to date reviews of effective care? *BMJ*: 1993; **307**: 1464.

27 Johnston ME, Langton KB, Haynes RB. A critical appraisal of research on the effects of computer-based decision support systems on clinical performance and patient outcome. *Ann Intern Med* 1994; **120**: 135–42.

28 Enkin M, Keirse MJNC, Renfrew MJ, Neilson JP. *A guide to effective care during pregnancy and childbirth*. 2nd ed. Oxford: Oxford University Press, 1995.

29 Chalmers I. Improving the quality and dissemination of reviews of clinical research. In: Lock S, ed. *The future of medical journals*. London: BMJ, 1991: 127–36.

30 Chalmers I, Enkin M, Keirse MJNC. Preparing and updating systematic reviews of randomized controlled trials of health care. *Milbank Q* 1993; **71**: 411–37.

31 The Cochrane Collaboration. *Introductory brochure*. Oxford: Cochrane Collaboration, 1993.

32 Lock S. *A question of balance: editorial peer review in medicine*. London: BMJ, 1986.

# Bibliography on the science of reviewing research

It occurred to us that it would be helpful to end this collection of papers about systematic reviews with a bibliography of publications relevant to the relatively young science of reviewing research. Like many good thoughts this one came close to the copy deadline. The bibliography has been compiled with much enthusiasm, little time, and much help from Jesse Berlin, Gord Guyatt, Les Irwig, Cynthia Mulrow, Arne Ohlsson, Ken Schulz, and Donna Stroup, who all made generous contributions at short notice. They deserve credit, but we must take responsibility for oversights and errors.

We hope that the bibliography will help those who are new to the science of reviewing to find additional material of interest, and those who are already immersed in it to find something new. The bibliography is not comprehensive and the inclusion criteria are not entirely clear. We have tried to include all the published empirical studies of methods used in reviews of which we are aware. We have also included methodological studies that are directly relevant to doing a review, such as empirical studies of the association between research methods and bias in randomised controlled trials.

To locate these references we have relied on our own file drawers, references lists, and contact with colleagues. We have included all of the books, conference proceedings, and special journal issues devoted to the topic of systematic reviews and meta-analysis of which we are aware; we have not listed separately their constituent chapters and articles. Among the articles we have listed we have included several of those introducing systematic reviews and meta-analysis to a wide audience, as well as others addressing specific issues of relevance. A number of general articles directed at specialist audiences have not been included.

Suggestions for additions to the bibliography are welcome. Please send copies of the articles to:

Andy Oxman
Department of Health Services Research
National Institute of Public Health
Geitmyrsveien 750
0462 Oslo
Norway

FAX: +47 22 04 25 95
E-mail: andrew.oxman@labmed.uio.no

The bibliography will be progressively developed and refined by contributors to the Cochrane Collaboration and others. Updated versions will be disseminated on disk with *The Cochrane Database of Systematic Reviews*, and these will also be made available through Internet using the FTP servers at the Canadian Cochrane Centre and the UK Cochrane Centre. Further information about the Cochrane Collaboration and how to access the FTP servers can be obtained by contacting any of the Cochrane centres listed below.

ANDY OXMAN, DOUGLAS ALTMAN, and IAIN CHALMERS

BIBLIOGRAPHY

# Further information about the Cochrane Collaboration can be obtained from:

**The Australasian Cochrane Centre**
Flinders Medical Centre
Bedford Park SA 5042
AUSTRALIA
Tel: +61-8-204-5255
Fax: +61-8-276-3305
E-mail: cochrane@flinders.edu.au

**The Baltimore Cochrane Center**
Department of Epidemiology
 and Preventive Medicine
University of Maryland
660 West Redwood Street
Baltimore
MD 21201-1596
USA
Tel: +1-410-706-5295
Fax: +1-410-706-8013
E-mail: cochrane@cosy.ab.umd.edu

**The Canadian Cochrane Centre**
Health Information Research Unit
McMaster University Medical
 Centre
1200 Main Street West
Hamilton
Ontario L8N 3Z5
CANADA
Tel: +1-905-525-9140 ext. 22311
Fax: +1-905-546-0401
E-mail: cochrane@mcmaster.ca
Anonymous FTP server:
ftp.cochrane.mcmaster.ca

**The Dutch Cochrane Centre**
Department of Clinical
 Epidemiology and Biostatistics
Academic Medical Centre
Meibergdreef 9
1105 AZ Amsterdam
Netherlands
Tel: +31-20-566-2723
Fax: +31-20-691-2683
E-mail: cochrane@amc.uva.nl

**The Italian Cochrane Centre**
Center for Health Care Research

Laboratory of Clinical
 Epidemiology
Mario Negri Institute
Via Eritrea 62
20157 Milano
ITALY
Tel: +39-2-39014-540
Fax: +39-2-33200-231
E-mail: cochrane@imimnvx.irfmn.
mnegri.it

**The Nordic Cochrane Centre**
Research and Development
 Secretariat
Rigshospitalet
9 Blegdamsvej
2100 Copenhagen Ø
DENMARK
Tel: +45-35-45-55-71
Fax: +45-35-45-65-28
E-mail: rifopg@pop.denet.dk

**The San Francisco Cochrane Center**
Institute for Health Policy Studies
University of California
1388 Sutter Street, 11th Floor
San Francisco
CA 94109
USA
Tel: +1-415-476-1067
Fax: +1-415-476-0705
E-mail: sfcc@sirius.com

**The UK Cochrane Centre**
NHS R&D Programme
Summertown Pavilion
Middle Way
Oxford OX2 7LG
UK
Tel: +44-1865-516300
Fax: +44-1865-516311
E-mail: general@cochrane.co.uk
Anonymous FTP server:
ftp.cochrane.co.uk

# BOOKS, CONFERENCE PROCEEDINGS AND SPECIAL ISSUES OF JOURNALS

Chalmers I, Altman DG (eds). *Systematic Reviews.* London: BMJ Publishing Group, 1995.

Chalmers TC (ed). *Data analysis for clinical medicine.* Rome: International University Press, 1988.

Cleary PD (ed). Effective care in pregnancy and childbirth. *Milbank Q* 1993; 71: 401–533.

Cook TC, Cooper H, Corday DS, *et al. Meta-analysis for explanation: A casebook.* New York: Russell Sage Foundation, 1993.

Cooper H, Hedges LV (eds). *The handbook of research synthesis.* New York: Russell Sage Foundation, 1993.

Cooper HM. *Integrating research. A guide for literature reviews.* 2nd edition. Newbury Park: Sage Publications, 1989.

Eddy DM, Hasselblad V, Shachter R. *Meta-analysis by the confidence profile method. The statistical synthesis of evidence.* Boston: Academic Press, 1992.

Everitt BS, Dunn G, Holford TR (eds). Meta-analysis. *Statistical Methods in Medical Research* 1993; 2: 117–92.

General Accounting Office. *Cross design synthesis: a new strategy for medical effectiveness research.* Washington, DC: GAO, 1992.

Glass GV, McGaw B, Smith M. *Meta-analysis in social research.* Newbury Park: Sage Publications, 1981.

Hedges LV, Olkin I. *Statistical methods for meta-analysis.* Orlando: Academic Press, 1985.

Hunter JE, Schmidt FL. *Methods of meta-analysis. Correcting error and bias in research findings.* Newbury Park: Sage Publications, 1990.

Jenicek M. *Méta-analyse en médecine: Évaluation et synthèse de l'information clinique et épidémiologique.* St-Hyacinthe: Edisem, 1987.

Light RJ (ed). *Evaluation studies review annual* (vol 8). Beverly Hills, CA: Sage, 1983.

Light RJ, Pillemer DB. *Summing up: The science of reviewing research.* Cambridge: Harvard University Press, 1984.

National Research Council. *On combining information: statistical issues and opportunities for research.* Washington, DC: National Academy of Sciences Press, 1992.

Noblit GW, Hare RD. Meta-ethnography: synthesizing qualitative studies. Newbury Park: Sage Publications, 1988.

Petitti DB. *Meta-analysis, decision analysis, and cost-effectiveness analysis. Methods for quantitative synthesis in medicine.* New York: Oxford University Press, 1994.

Rosenthal R. Meta-analytic procedures for social research. Revised edition. Newbury Park: Sage Publications, 1991.

Sackett DL, Oxman AD (eds). *The Cochrane Collaboration handbook.* Oxford: Cochrane Collaboration, 1994.

Spitzer WO (ed). *The Potsdam international consultation on meta-analysis. J Clin Epidemiol* 1995; 48: 1–172.

Wachter KW, Straf ML (eds). *The future of meta-analysis*. New York: Russell Sage Foundation, 1990.

Warren KS, Mosteller F (eds). *Doing more good than harm: the evaluation of health care interventions*. The Third L.W. Frohlich Awards Conference in the Series Science and the Human Prospect. *Ann NY Acad Sci* 1993: 703.

Wolf FM. *Meta-Analysis. Quantitative methods for research synthesis*. Series: Quantitative applications in the social sciences No 59. Beverly Hills, CA: Sage Publications, 1986.

Yeaton WH, Wortman PM (eds). *Issues in data synthesis*. San Francisco: Jossey-Bass, 1984.

Yusuf S, Simon R, Ellenberg S (eds). Proceedings of 'methodologic issues in overviews of randomized clinical trials'. *Stat Med* 1987; **6**: 217–409.

# ARTICLES

Each paper in the following list has been classified using one or more of the following codes:

Gen: General articles about the science of reviewing research
Id: Identification and selection of trials, publication and other 'selection' biases, and registers of trials
Qual: Assessment of methodological quality, data collection, and reviews using individual patient data
M-A: Data synthesis (meta-analysis)
Rep: Conclusions and reporting

Abel UR, Edler L. A pitfall in the meta-analysis of hazard ratios. *Controlled Clin Trials* 1988; **9**: 149–51. [M-A]

Abramson JH. Meta-analysis: a review of pros and cons. *Public Health Rev* 1990; **18**: 1–47. [Gen]

Adams CE, Lefebvre C, Chalmers I. Bugs discovered during SilverPlatter MEDLINE searches for RCTs. *Lancet* 1992; **340**: 915–6. [Id]

Adams CE, Power A, Frederick K, Lefebvre C. An investigation of the adequacy of MEDLINE searches for randomized controlled trials (RCTs) of the effects of mental health care. *Psychol Med* 1994; **24**: 741–8. [Id]

Altman DG, Doré CJ. Randomisation and baseline comparisons in clinical trials. *Lancet* 1990; **335**: 149–53. [Qual]

Andersen JW, Harrington D. Meta-analyses need new publication standards. *J Clin Oncol* 1992; **10**: 878–80. [Rep]

Anonymous. *ASA/EPA Conferences on interpretation of environmental data: II statistical issues in combining environmental studies*. Washington DC: EPA, 1986. [M-A]

Antman EM, Lau J, Kupelnick B, Mosteller F, Chalmers TC. A comparison of results of meta-analyses of randomized control trials and recommendations of clinical experts. *JAMA* 1992; **268**: 240–8. [Gen]

Bailey KR. Generalizing the results of randomized clinical trials. *Controlled Clin Trials* 1994; **15**: 15–23. [Rep]

Baissel JP, Ad Hoc Working Party of the International Collaborative Group on Clinical Trial Registries. Position paper and consensus recommendation on clinical trial registraties. *Clinical Trials Meta-Anal* 1993; **28**: 255–66 [Id]

Bangert-Drowns RL. Review of developments in meta-analytic method. *Psychol Bull* 1986; **99**: 388–99. [Gen]

Bausell RB. After the meta-analytic revolution. *Evaluation and the Health Professions* 1993; **16**: 3–12. [Gen]

Begg CB, Berlin JA. Publication bias: a problem in interpreting medical data. *Journal of the Royal Statistical Society* A 1988; **151**: 419–63. [Id]

Begg CB, Berlin JA. Publication bias and dissemination of clinical research. *J Natl Cancer Inst* 1989; **81**: 107–15. [Id]

Begg CB, Pilote L. A model for incorporating historical controls into a meta-analysis. *Biometrics* 1991; **47**: 899–906. [M-A]

Berlin JA. Meta-analysis. In: Strom BL (ed). *Pharmacoepidemiology*. John Wiley and Sons, 1994. [Gen]

Berlin JA, Begg CB, Louis TA. An assessment of publication bias using a sample of published clinical trials. *Journal of the American Statistical Association* 1989; **84**: 381–92. [Id]

Berlin JA, Laird NM, Sacks HS, Chalmers TC. A comparison of statistical methods for combining event rates from clinical trials. *Stat Med* 1989; **8**: 141–51. [M-A]

Berlin JA, Longnecker MP, Greenland S. Meta-analysis of epidemiologic dose-response data. *Epidemiology* 1993; **6**: 218–28. [M-A]

Bernstein F. The retrieval of randomized clinical trials in liver diseases from the medical literature: Manual versus MEDLARS searches. *Controlled Clin Trials* 1988; **9**: 23–31. [Id]

Bero LA, Glantz SA, Rennie D. Publication bias and public health policy on environmental tobacco smoke. *JAMA*; **272**: 133–6. [Id]

Bero LA, Rennie D. Influences on the quality of published drug studies. *International Journal of Technology Assessment in Health Care*. (In Press) [Qual]

Bobbio M, Demichelis B, Giustetto G. Completeness of reporting trial results: effect on physicians' willingness to prescribe. *Lancet* 1994; **343**: 1209–11. [Rep]

Boissel JP, Ad Hoc Working Party of the International Collaborative Group on Clinical Trial Registries. Position paper and consensus recommendation on clinical trial registries. *Clin Trials Meta-Anal* 1993; **28**: 255–66. [Id]

Boissel JP, Blanchard J, Panak E, Payrieux JC, Sacks H. Considerations for the meta-analysis of randomized clinical trials: summary of a panel discussion. *Controlled Clin Trials* 1989; **10**: 254–81. [Gen]

Bracken MB. Statistical methods for analysis of effects of treatment in overviews of randomized trials. In: Sinclair JC, Bracken MB (eds). *Effective care of the newborn infant*. Oxford: Oxford University Press, 1992: 13-8. [M-A]

Breslow NE, Day NE. *Analysis of case-control studies. Statistical methods in cancer research* (Vol 1). Lyon: International Agency for Research on Cancer, 1980: 122-59. [M-A]

Buffler PA. The evaluation of negative epidemiologic studies: the importance of all available evidence in risk characterisation. *Regulatory Toxicology and Pharmacology* 1989; 9: 34–43. [M-A]

Bulpitt CJ. Meta-analysis. *Lancet* 1988; ii: 93–4. [Gen]

Buyse ME, Ryan LM. Issues of efficiency in combining proportions of deaths from several trials. *Stat Med* 1987; 6: 565–76. [M-A]

Campbell DT, Stanley JC. *Experimental and quasi-experimental designs for research.* Chicago: Rand McNally College Publishing Company, 1966. [Qual]

Carlin JB. Meta-analysis for 2×2 tables: a Bayesian approach. *Stat Med* 1992; 11: 141-51. [M-A]

Chalmers I. Under-reporting research is scientific misconduct. *JAMA* 1990; 263: 1405–8. [Id]

Chalmers I. Improving the quality and dissemination of reviews of clinical research. In: Lock S (ed). *The future of medical journals. In commemoration of 150 years of the British Medical Journal.* London: BMJ Publishing Group, 1991 127–46. [Gen]

Chalmers I. Can meta-analyses be trusted? *Lancet* 1991; 338: 1464–5. [Gen]

Chalmers I. Publication bias. *Lancet* 1993; 342: 1116. [Id]

Chalmers I, Haynes B. Reporting, updating, and correcting systematic reviews of the effects of health care. *BMJ* 1994; 309: 862-5. [Gen]

Chalmers I, Dickersin K, Chalmers TC. Getting to grips with Archie Cochrane's agenda: a register of all randomized controlled trials. *BMJ* 1992; 305: 786–8. [Id]

Chalmers I, Hetherington J, Elbourne D, Keirse MJNC, Enkin M. Materials and methods used in synthesizing evidence to evaluate the effects of care during pregnancy and childbirth. In: Chalmers I, Enkin M, Keirse MJNC (eds). *Effective care in pregnancy and childbirth.* Oxford: Oxford University Press, 1989, 39–65. [Gen, Qual]

Chalmers I, Hetherington J, Newdick M, Mutch L, Grant A, Enkin M, Enkin E, Dickersin K. The Oxford Database of Perinatal Trials: developing a register of published reports of controlled trials. *Controlled Clin Trials* 1986; 7: 306–24. [Id]

Chalmers TC. Problems induced by meta-analyses. *Stat Med* 1991; 10: 971–80. [Gen]

Chalmers TC, Berrier J, Sacks HS, Levin H, Reitman D, Nagalingam R. Meta-analysis of clinical trials as a scientific discipline. II: replicate variability and comparison of studies that agree and disagree. *Stat Med* 1987; 6: 733–44. [Gen]

Chalmers TC, Celano P, Sacks HS, Smith H. Bias in treatment assignment in controlled clinical trials. *N Engl J Med* 1983; 309: 1358–61. [Qual]

Chalmers TC, Frank CS, Reitman D. Minimizing the three stages of publication bias. *JAMA* 1990; 263: 1392–5. [Id]

Chalmers TC, Koff RS, Grady GF. A note on fatality in serum hepatitis. *Gastroenterology* 1965; 49: 22–6. [Id]

Chalmers TC, Levin H, Sacks HS, Reitman D, Berrier J, Nagalingam R. Meta-analysis of clinical trials as a scientific discipline. I: control of bias and comparison with large co-operative trials. *Stat Med* 1987; 6: 315–25. [Gen]

Chalmers TC, Matta RJ, Smith H Jr, Kunzler AM. Evidence favoring the use of anticoagulants in the hospital phase of acute myocardial infarction. *N Engl J Med* 1977; 297: 1091–6. [Qual]

Cho MK, Bero LA. Instruments for assessing the quality of drug studies published in the medical literature. *JAMA* 1994; 272: 101–4. [Qual]

Clarke M. Searching Medline for randomised trials. *BMJ* 1993; 307: 565. [Id]

Clarke MJ, Stewart LA. Obtaining data from randomised trials: how much do we need in order to perform reliable and informative metal-analyses? *BMJ* 1994; 309: 1007–10. [Qual]

Cochran WG. Problems arising in the analysis of a series of similar experiments. *Journal of the Royal Statistical Society* (Suppl) 1937; 4: 102–18. [M-A]

Cochran WG. The combination of estimates from different experiments. *Biometrics* 1954; 3: 101–29. [M-A]

Colditz GA, Miller JN, Mosteller F. How study design affects outcomes in comparisons of therapy. I: medical. *Stat Med* 1989; 8: 441–54.

Cook DJ, Guyatt GH, Laupacis A, Sackett DL. Rules of evidence and clinical recommendations in the use of antithrombotic agents. Antithrombotic Therapy Consensus Conference. *Chest* 1992; 102: 305S–11S. [Rep]

Cook DJ, Guyatt GH, Ryan G, *et al*. Should unpublished data be included in meta-analyses? *JAMA* 1993; 269: 2749–53. [Id]

Cook TD, Leviton LC. Reviewing the literature: a comparison of traditional methods with meta-analysis. *Journal of Personality* 1980; 48: 448–71. [Gen]

Cooper H, Ribble RG. Influences on the outcome of literature searches for integrative research reviews. *Knowledge* 1989; 10: 179–201. [Id]

Cooper HM, Rosenthal R. Statistical versus traditional procedures for summarizing research findings. *Psychol Bull* 1980; 87: 442–449. [Gen, M-A]

Counsell C, Fraser H. Identifying relevant studies for systematic reviews. *BMJ* 1995; 310: 126. [Id]

Counsell CE, Clarke MJ, Slattery J, Sandercock PAG. The miracle of DICE therapy for acute stroke: fact or fictional product of subgroup analysis? *BMJ* 1994; 309: 1677–81. [Rep]

Counsell CE, Fraser H, Sandercock PAG. Archie Cochrane's challenge: can periodically updated reviews of all randomised controlled trials relevant to neurology and neurosurgery be produced? *J Neurol Neurosurg Psychiatry* 1994; 57: 529–33. [Id]

Davidson RA. Source of funding and outcome of clinical trials. *J Gen Intern Med* 1986; 1: 155–8. [Id]

Dear KBG, Begg CB. An approach for assessing publication bias prior to performing a meta-analysis. *Statistical Science* 1992; 7: 237–45. [Id]

DerSimonian R, Laird N. Meta-analysis in clinical trials. *Controlled Clin Trials* 1986; **7**: 177–88. [M-A]

Detsky AS, Naylor CD, O'Rourke K, McGeer AJ, L'Abbé KA. Incorporating variations in the quality of individual randomized trials into meta-analysis. *J Clin Epidemiol* 1992; **45**: 255–65. [Qual]

Dickersin K. Report from the panel on the case for registers of clinical trials. *Controlled Clin Trials* 1988; **9**: 76–81. [Id]

Dickersin K. The existence of publication bias and risk factors for its occurrence *JAMA* 1990; **263**: 1385–9. [Id]

Dickersin K. Keeping posted. Why register clinical trials? - revisited. *Controlled Clin Trials* 1992; **13**: 170–7. [Id]

Dickersin K, Berlin JA. Meta-analysis: state-of-the-science. *Epidemiol Rev* 1992; **14**: 154–76. [Gen]

Dickersin K, Chan S, Chalmers TC, Sacks HS, Smith H. Publication bias and clinical trials. *Controlled Clin Trials* 1987; **8**: 343–53. [Id]

Dickersin K, Hewitt P, Mutch L, Chalmers I, Chalmers TC. Comparison of MEDLINE searching with a perinatal trials database. *Controlled Clin Trials* 1985; **6**: 306–17. [Id]

Dickersin K, Higgins K, Meinert CL. Identification of meta-analyses: the need for standard terminology. *Controlled Clin Trials* 1990; **11**: 52–66. [Gen]

Dickersin K, Min YI. NIH clinical trials and publication bias. *Online J Curr Clin Trials* [serial online] 1993; Doc No 50: 4967 words; 53 paragraphs. [Id]

Dickersin K, Min YI, Meinert CL. Factors influencing publication of research results: follow-up of applications submitted to two institutional review boards. *JAMA* 1992; **263**: 374–8. [Id]

Dickersin K, Scherer R, Lefebvre C. Identifying relevant studies for systematic reviews. *BMJ* 1994; **309**: 1286–91. [Id]

Duffy SW, Rohan TE, Altman DG. A method for combining matched and unmatched binary data. *Am J Epidemiol* 1989; **130**: 371–8. [M-A]

Early Breast Cancer Trialists' Collaborative Group. Statistical Methods. In: *Treatment of early breast cancer.* Vol 1. Worldwide evidence 1985-1990. Oxford: Oxford University Press, 1990: 13-8. [M-A]

Easterbrook PJ. Directory of registries of clinical trials. *Stat Med* 1992; **11**: 345–423. [Id]

Easterbrook PJ, Berlin JA, Gopalan R, Matthews DR. Publication bias in clinical research. *Lancet* 1991; **337**: 867–72. [Id]

Eddy DM. Anatomy of a decision. *JAMA* 1990; **263**: 441–3. [Rep]

Eddy DM, Hasselblad V, Schachter R. An introduction to a Bayesian method for meta-analysis: the confidence profile method. *Medical Decision Making* 1990; **10**: 15–23. [M-A]

Emerson JD, Burdick E, Hoaglin DC, Mosteller F, Chalmers TC. An empirical study of the possible relation of treatment differences to quality scores in controlled randomized clinical trials. *Controlled Clin Trials* 1990; **11**: 339–52. [Qual]

Eysenck HJ. Meta-analysis and its problems. *BMJ* 1994; **309**: 789–92. [M-A]

Feinstein AR. *Clinical epidemiology: the architecture of clinical research.* Philadelphia: Saunders, 1985. [Qual]

Felson DT. Bias in meta-analytic research. *J Clin Epidemiol* 1992; 45: 885–92. [Gen]

Fleiss JL, Gross AJ. Meta-analysis in epidemiology, with special reference to studies of the association between exposure to environmental tobacco smoke and lung cancer: a critique. *J Clin Epidemiol* 1991; 44: 127–39. [M-A]

Follmann D, Elliott P, Suh I, Cutler J. Variance imputation for overviews of clinical trials with continuous response. *J Clin Epidemiol* 1992; 45: 769–73. [M-A]

Friedenreich CM. Methods for pooled analyses of epidemiologic studies. *Epidemiology* 1993; 4: 295–302. [Gen]

Friedenreich CM, Brant RF, Riboli E. Influence of methodologic factors in a pooled analysis of 13 case-control studies of colorectal cancer and dietary fiber. *Epidemiology* 1994; 5: 66–79. [Qual]

Galbraith RF. A note on graphical presentation of estimated odds ratios from several clinical trials. *Stat Med* 1988; 7: 889–94. [M-A]

Gelber RD, Goldhirsh A. From the overview to the patient: how to interpret meta-analysis data. *Recent Results in Cancer Research* 1993; 127: 167–76. [Rep]

Geller NL, Scher HI, Parmar MKB, Dalesio O, Kaye S. Can we combine available data to evaluate the effects of neoadjuvant chemotherapy for invasive bladder cancer? *Semin Oncol* 1990; 17: 628–34. [Id]

Glass GV. Primary, secondary, and meta-analysis of research. *Educational Researcher* 1976; 5: 3–8. [Gen]

Goodman SN. Meta-analysis and evidence. *Controlled Clin Trials* 1989; 10: 188–204, 435 (erratum). [Gen]

Goodman SN. Have you ever meta-analysis you didn't like? *Ann Intern Med* 1991; 114: 244–6. [Gen]

Gøtzsche PC. Reference bias in reports of drug trials. *BMJ* 1987; 295: 654–6. [Id]

Gøtzsche PC. Methodology and overt and hidden bias in reports of 196 double-blind trials of nonsteroidal antiinflammatory drugs in rheumatoid arthritis. *Controlled Clin Trials* 1989; 10: 31–56. [Qual]

Gøtzsche P. Patients' preference in indomethacin trials: an overview. *Lancet* 1989; 1: 88–90. [Qual]

Gøtzsche P. Multiple publication of reports of drug trials. *Eur J Clin Pharmacol* 1989; 36: 429–32. [Id]

Gøtzsche P. Meta-analysis of NSAIDs: contribution of drugs, doses, trial designs, and meta-analytic techniques. *Scand J Rheumatol* 1993; 22: 255–60. [Qual, M-A]

Gøtzsche PC. Sensitivity of effect variables in rheumatoid arthritis: a meta-analysis of 130 placebo controlled nsaid trials. *J Clin Epidemiol* 1990; 43: 1313–8. [Qual]

Gøtzsche PC, Lange B. Comparison of search strategies for recalling doubleblind trials from MEDLINE. *Dan Med Bull* 1991; 38: 47–68. [Id]

Gøtzsche PC, Podenphant J, Olesen M, Halberg P. Meta-analysis of second-line antirheumatic drugs: sample size bias and uncertain benefit. *J Clin Epidemiol* 1992; **45**: 587–94. [M-A]

Greenland S. Interpretation and estimation of summary ratios under heterogeneity. *Stat Med* 1982; **1**: 217–27. [Rep]

Greenland S. Quantitative methods in the review of epidemiologic literature. *Epidemiol Rev* 1987; **9**: 1–30. [M-A]

Greenland S. Can meta-analysis be salvaged? *Am J Epidemiol* 1994; **140**: 783–7. [Gen]

Greenland S. Invited commentary: a critical look at some popular meta-analytic methods. *Am J Epidemiol* 1994; **140**: 290–6. [Gen]

Greenland S, Longnecker MP. Methods for trend estimation from summarized dose-response data, with applications to meta-analysis. *Am J Epidemiol* 1992; **135**: 1301–9. [M-A]

Greenland S, Salvan A. Bias in the one-step (Peto) method for pooling study results. *Stat Med* 1990; **9**: 247–52. [M-A]

Harlan WR. Creating an NIH clinical trials registry: a user-friendly approach to health care. *JAMA* 1994; **271**: 1729. [Id]

Hauck WW. A comparative study of conditional maximum likelihood estimation of a common odds ratio. *Biometrics* 1984; **40**: 1117–23. [M-A]

Haynes RB. Clinical review articles: should be as scientific as the articles they review. *BMJ* 1992; **304**: 330–1. [Gen]

Haynes RB, Mulrow CD, Huth EJ, Altman DG, Gardner MJ. More informative abstracts revisited. *Ann Intern Med* 1990; **113**: 69–76. [Rep]

Hedges LV. How hard is hard science, how soft is soft science? The empirical cumulativeness of research. *American Psychologist* 1987; **42**: 443–55. [Gen]

Hedges LV. Modelling publication selection effects in meta-analysis. *Statistical Science* 1992; **7**: 246–55. [Id]

Hemminki E. Study of information submitted by drug companies to licensing authorities. *BMJ* 1980; **i**: 833–6. [Id]

Henry DA, Wilson A. Meta-analysis: part 1: an assessment of its aims, validity and reliability. *Med J Aust* 1992; **156**: 31–8. [Gen]

Hetherington J, Dickersin K, Chalmers I, Meinert CL. Retrospective and prospective identification of unpublished controlled trials: lessons from a survey of obstetricians and pediatricians. *Pediatrics* 1989; **84**: 374–80. [Id]

Hill AB. *Principles of medical statistics.* 9th ed. London: Lancet, 1971: 312–20. [Rep]

Hofmans EA. The results of a MEDLINE search. The accessibility of research on the effectiveness of acupuncture II. *Huisarts Wet* 1990; **33**: 103–6. [Id]

Huth EJ. Needed: review article with more scientific rigor. *Ann Intern Med* 1987; **106**: 470–1. [Gen]

Irwig L, Tosteson NA, Gatsonis C, Lau J, Colditz G, Chalmers TC, Mosteller F. Guidelines for meta-analyses evaluating diagnostic tests. *Ann Intern Med* 1994; **120**: 667–76. [Gen]

Iyengar S, Greenhouse JB. Selection models and the file drawer problem. *Statistical Science* 1988; **3**: 109–35. [Id]

Jackson GB. Methods for integrative reviews. *Review of Educational Research* 1980; **50**: 438-60. [Gen]

Jadad AR, McQuay HJ. A highyield strategy to identify randomized controlled trials for systematic reviews. *Online J Curr Clin Trials* [serial online] 1993; Doc No 33: 3973 words; 39 paragraphs. [Id]

Jadad AR, McQuay HJ. Be systematic in your searching. *BMJ* 1993; **307**: 66. [Id]

Jenicek M. Meta-analysis in medicine, where we are and where we want to go. *J Clin Epidemiol* 1989; **42**: 35–44. [Gen]

Jones DR. Meta-analysis: weighing the evidence. *Stat Med* 1995; **14**: 137–49. [Gen]

Kirpalani H, Schmidt B, McKibbon KA, Haynes RB, Sinclair JC. Searching MEDLINE for randomized clinical trials involving care of the newborn. *Pediatrics* 1989; **83**: 543–6. [Id]

Kleijnen J, Knipschild P. The comprehensiveness of MEDLINE and EMBASE computer searches. Searches for controlled trials of homeopathy, ascorbic acid for common cold and ginkgo biloba for cerebral insufficiency and intermittent claudication. *Pharm Weekbl [Sci]* 1992; **14**: 316–20. [Id]

Knipschild P. Systematic reviews: some examples. *BMJ* 1994; **309**: 719–21. [Gen]

Koren G, Graham K, Shear H, Einarson T. Bias against the null hypothesis: the reproductive hazards of cocaine. *Lancet* 1989; ii: 1440–2. [Id]

L'Abbé KA, Detsky AS, O'Rourke K. Meta-analysis in clinical research. *Ann Intern Med* 1987; **107**: 224–33. [Gen]

Laird NM, Mosteller F. Some statistical methods for combining experimental results. *Int J Technol Assess Health Care* 1990; **6**: 5–30. [M-A]

Lancet. Making clinical trialists register. *Lancet* 1991; **338**: 244–5. [Id]

Lau J, Antman EM, Jimenez-Silva J, Kupelnick B, Mosteller F, Chalmers TC. Cumulative meta-analysis of therapeutic trials for myocardial infarction. *N Engl J Med* 1992; **327**: 248–54. [M-A]

Laupacis A, Sackett DL, Roberts RS. An assessment of clinically useful measures of the consequences of treatment. *N Engl J Med* 1988; **318**: 1728–33. [M-A, Rep]

Lee YJ, Ellenberg JH, Hirtz DG, Nelson KB. Analysis of clinical trials by treatment actually received: is it really an option? *Stat Med* 1991; **10**: 1595–1605. [Qual]

Leizorovicz A, Haugh MC, Boissel JP. Meta-analysis and multiple publication of clinical trial reports. *Lancet* 1992; **340**: 1102-3. [Id]

Li Z, Begg CB. Random effects models for combining results from controlled and uncontrolled studies in a meta-analysis. *Journal of the American Statistical Association* 1994; **89**: 1523–7. [M-A]

Light RJ, Smith PV. Accumulating evidence: procedures for resolving contradictions among different research studies. *Harvard Educational Review* 1971; **41**: 429–71. [Gen]

BIBLIOGRAPHY

Linde K, Melchart F, Jonas WB. Durchführung und Interpretation systematischer Übersichtsarbeiten kontrollierter Studien in der Komplementärmedizin. *Separata aus Forschende Komplementärmedizin* 1994; **1**: 8–16. [Gen]

Littenberg B, Moses LE. Estimating diagnostic accuracy from multiple conflicting reports. *Medical Decision Making* 1993; **13**: 313–21. [Gen]

Lund T. Some metrical issues with meta-analysis of therapy effects. *Scand J Psychol* 1988; **29**: 1–8. [M-A]

Mahoney MJ. Bias, controversy, and abuse in the study of the scientific publication system. *Science, Technology, and Human Values* 1990; **15**: 50–5. [Id]

McKinlay SM. The effect of nonzero second-order interaction on combined estimators of the odds ratio. *Biometrika* 1978; **65**: 191–202. [M-A]

Meinert CL. *Clinical trials: design, conduct and analysis.* Oxford: Oxford University Press, 1986. [Qual]

Meinert CL. Toward prospective registration of clinical trials. *Controlled Clin Trials* 1988; **9**: 1–5. [Id]

Meinert CL. Meta-analysis: science or religion? *Controlled Clin Trials* 1989; **10**: 257S-63S. [Gen]

Messori A, Rampazzo R. Meta-analysis of clinical trials based on censored end-points: simplified theory and implementation of the statistical algorithms on a microcomputer. *Comput Meth Prog Biomed* 1993; **40**: 261–7.

Mi J. Notes on the MLE of correlation-coefficient in meta analysis. *Communications in Statistics, Theory and Methods* 1990; **19**: 2035-52. [M-A]

Midgette AS, Stukel TA, Littenberg B. A meta-analytic method for summarizing diagnostic test performance: receiver-operating-characteristic summary point estimates *Medical Decision Making* 1993; **13**: 253–7. [M-A]

Miller JN, Colditz GA, Mosteller F. How study design affects outcomes in comparisons of therapy. II: surgical. *Stat Med* 1989; **8**: 455–66. [Qual]

Moses L, Littenberg B, Shapiro D. Combining independent studies of a diagnostic test into a summary ROC curve: data-analytic approaches and some additional considerations. *Stat Med* 1993; **12**: 1293–316. [M-A]

Mosteller F. Using meta-analysis for research synthesis: pooling data from several studies. In: Ingelfinger JA, Mosteller F, Thibodeau LA, Ware JH. *Biostatistics in clinical medicine*, 3rd ed. New York: McGraw-Hill, 1994: 332–60. [Gen]

Mosteller F, Chalmers TC. Some progress and problems in meta-analysis of clinical trials. *Statistical Science* 1992; **7**: 227–236. [Gen]

Mosteller F, Gilbert JP, McPeek B. Reporting standards and research strategies for controlled trials: agenda for the editor. *Controlled Clinical Trials* 1980; **1**: 37–58. [Qual]

Mulrow CD. The medical review article: state of the science. *Ann Intern Med* 1987; **106**: 485–8. [Gen]

Mulrow CD. Rationale for systematic reviews. *BMJ* 1994; **309**: 597–9. [Gen]

Mulrow CD, Thacker SB, Pugh JA. A proposal for more informative abstracts of review articles. *Ann Intern Med* 1988; **108**: 613–5. [Gen]

Munoz A, Rosner B. Power and sample size for a collection of $2 \times 2$ tables. *Biometrics* 1984; **40**: 995–1004. [M-A]

National Library of Medicine. *List of journals indexed in "Index Medicus"*. Bethesda: National Library of Medicine, 1994. [Id]

Naylor CD. Two cheers for meta-analysis: problems and opportunities in aggregating results of clinical trials. *Can Med Assoc J* 1988; **138**: 891–5. [Gen]

Naylor CD, Llewellyn-Thomas HA. Can there be a more patient-centred approach to determining clinically important effect sizes for randomized treatment trials? *J Clin Epidemiol* 1994; **47**: 787–95. [Rep]

Nylenna M, Riis P, Karlsson Y. Multiple blinded reviews of the same two manuscripts: effects of referee characteristics and publication language. *JAMA* 1994; **272**: 149–51. [Id]

O'Rourke K. Detsky AS. Second thoughts: meta-analysis in medical research: strong encouragement for higher quality in individual research efforts. *J Clin Epidemiol* 1989; **42**: 1021–6. [Qual]

Olkin I. Reconcilable differences. *The Sciences* 1992 (July/August): 30–36. [Gen]

*Online Databases in the Medical and Life Sciences*. New York: Cuadra/Elsevier, 1987. [Id]

Ottenbacher K. Impact of random assignment on study outcome: an empirical examination. *Controlled Clin Trials* 1992; **13**: 50–61. [Qual]

Oxman AD. Checklists for review articles. *BMJ* 1994; **309**: 648–51. [Gen]

Oxman AD, Cook DJ, Guyatt GH, for the Evidence-Based Medicine Working Group. Users' guides to the medical literature, VI: how to use an overview. *JAMA* 1994; **272**: 1367–71. [Gen]

Oxman AD, Guyatt GH. Guidelines for reading literature reviews. *Can Med Assoc J* 1988; **138**: 697–703. [Gen]

Oxman AD, Guyatt GH. Validation of an index of the quality of review articles. *J Clin Epidemiol* 1991; **11**: 1271–8. [Gen]

Oxman AD, Guyatt GH. A consumer's guide to subgroup analyses. *Ann Intern Med* 1992; **116**: 78–84. [Rep]

Oxman AD, Guyatt GH, Singer J, Goldsmith CH, Hutchison BG, Milner RA, Streiner DL. Agreement among reviewers of review articles. *J Clin Epidemiol* 1991; **44**: 91–8. [Gen]

Paul SR, Donner AP. A comparison of tests of homogeneity of odds ratios in K $2 \times 2$ tables. *Stat Med* 1989; **8**: 1455–68. [M-A]

Petitti DB. Of babies and bathwater. *Am J Epidemiol* 1994; **140**: 770–82. [Gen]

Peto R, Pike MC, Armitage P, Breslow NE, Cox DR, Howard SV, Mantel N, McPherson K, Peto J, Smith PG. Design and analysis of randomized clinical trials requiring prolonged observation of each patient. II: Analysis and examples. *Br J Cancer* 1977; **35**: 1–39. [M-A]

Pignon JP, Arriagada R. Meta-analysis. *Lancet* 1993; **341**: 418–22. [Qual]

BIBLIOGRAPHY

Pignon JP, Poynard T. Méta-analyse des essais thérapeutiques. *Gastroenterol Clin Biol* 1991; **15**: 229–38. [Gen]

Pignon JP, Arriagada R. Meta-analyses of randomized clinical trials: how to improve their quality. *Lung Cancer* 1994; **10**: S135–41. [Gen]

Pocock SJ. *Clinical trials: a practical approach.* Chichester: Wiley, 1983. [Qual]

Pocock SJ, Hughes MD. Estimation issues in clinical trials and overviews. *Stat Med* 1990; **9**: 657–71. [Id]

Poynard T, Conn HO. The retrieval of randomized clinical trials in liver disease from the medical literature. A comparison of MEDLARS and manual methods. *Controlled Clin Trials* 1985; **6**: 271–9. [Id]

Raghunathan TE, Yoichi II. Analysis of binary data from a multicentre clinical trial. *Biometrika* 1993; **80**: 127–39. [M-A]

Ravnskov U. Cholesterol lowering trials in coronary heart disease: frequency of citation and outcome. *BMJ* 1992; **305**: 15–19. [Id]

Rifat SL. Graphic representations of effect estimates: an example from a meta-analytic review. *J Clin Epidemiol* 1990; **43**: 1267–71. [Rep]

Robins J, Greenland S, Breslow NE. A general estimator for the variance of the Mantel-Haenszel odds ratio. *Am J Epidemiol* 1986; **124**: 719–23. [M-A]

Rochon PA, Gurwitz JH, Cheung CM, Hayes HA, Chalmers TC. Evaluating the quality of articles published in journal supplements compared with the quality of those published in the parent journal. *JAMA* 1994; **272**: 108–13. [Qual]

Rosendaal FR, Van Everdingen JJE. Cumulatieve metanalyse als ultime waarheid. *Ned Tidschr Geneeskd* 1993; **137**: 1591–4. [Gen]

Sackett DL, Cook RJ. Understanding clinical trials. *BMJ* 1994; **309**: 755–6. [Rep]

Sacks H, Chalmers TC, Smith H. Randomized versus historical controls for clinical trials. *Am J Med* 1982; **72**: 233–40. [Qual]

Sacks HS, Berrier J, Reitman D, Ancona-Berk VA, Chalmers TC. Meta-analyses of randomized controlled trials. *N Engl J Med* 1987; **316**: 450–5. [Gen]

Sacks HS, Berrier J, Reitman D, Pagano D, Chalmers TC. Meta-analyses of randomized control trials: an update of the quality and methodology. In: Bailar JC, Mosteller F (eds). *Medical uses of statistics.* 2nd ed. Boston: NEJM Books, 1992: 427–42. [Gen]

Scherer RW, Dickersin K, Kaplan E. The accessible biomedical literature represents a fraction of all studies in a field. In: Weeks RA, Kinser DL (eds). *Editing the refereed scientific journal: practical, political, and ethical issues.* New York: IEEE Press, 1994: 120–5. [Id]

Scherer RW, Dickersin K, Langenberg P. Full publication of results initially presented in abstracts: a meta-analysis. *JAMA* 1994: **272**: 158–62. [Id]

Schneider B. Analysis of clinical trial outcomes: alternative approaches to subgroup analysis. *Controlled Clin Trials* 1989; **10**: 176S–86S. [M-A]

Schoolman HM. Retrieving information on clinical trial methodology. *Clin Pharmacol Ther* 1979; **25**: 758–60. [Id]

Schulz KF, Altman DG. *Statistical methods for data synthesis. Cochrane Workshop Report*. Oxford: UK Cochrane Centre, 1993. [M-A]

Schulz KF, Chalmers I, Grimes DA, Altman DG. Assessing the quality of randomization from reports of controlled trials published in obstetrics and gynecology journals. *JAMA* 1994; 272: 125–8. [Qual]

Schulz KF, Chalmers I, Hayes RJ, Altman DG. Empirical evidence of bias: dimensions of methodological quality associated with estimates of treatment effects in controlled trials. *JAMA* 1995; 273: 408–12. [Qual]

Shapiro S. Meta-analysis/shmeta-analysis. *Am J Epidemiol* 1994; 140: 771–8, 788-91. [Gen]

Silagy C. Developing a register of randomized controlled trials in primary care. *BMJ* 1993; 306: 897–900. [Id]

Silagy CA, Jewell D. Review of 39 years of randomized controlled trials in the *British Journal of General Practice.Br J Gen Pract* 1994; 44: 359–63. [Id]

Silagy CA, Jewell D, Mant D. An analysis of randomized controlled trials published in the US family medicine literature, 1987–1991. *J Fam Pract* 1994; 39: 236–42. [Id]

Simes RJ. Publication bias: the case for an international registry of clinical trials. *J Clin Oncol* 1986; 4: 1529–41. [Id]

Simes RJ. Confronting publication bias: a cohort design for meta-analysis. *Stat Med* 1987; 6: 11–29. [Id]

Sinclair JC, Bracken MB. Clinically useful measures of effect in binary analyses of randomized trials. *J Clin Epidemiol* 1994; 47: 881–9. [Rep]

Smith ML. Publication bias and meta-analysis. *Evaluation in Education* 1980; 4: 22–4. [Id]

Solari ME, Wheatley D. A method of combining the results of several clinical trials. *Clinical Trials Journal* 1966; 3: 537–45. [M-A]

Solomon MJ, Laxamana A, Devore L, McLeod RS. Randomized controlled trials in surgery. *Surgery* 1994; 115: 707–12. [Id]

Søreide E, Steen PA. Dangers of review articles. *BMJ* 1993; 306: 66–7. [Gen]

Spector TD, Thompson SG. The potential and limitations of meta-analysis. *J Epidemiol Commun Health* 1991; 45: 89–92. [Gen]

Standards of Reporting Trials Group. A proposal for structured reporting of randomized controlled trials. *JAMA* 1994; 272: 1926–31. [Qual]

Sternsward J. Decreased survival related to irradiation postoperatively in early operable breast cancer. *Lancet* 1974; ii: 1285–6. [Gen]

Stewart LA, Parmar MKB. Meta-analysis of the literature or of individual patient data: is there a difference? *Lancet* 1993; 341: 418–22. [Qual]

Stock WA, Okun MA, Haring MJ, Miller W, Ceurvost RW. Rigor in data synthesis: a case study of reliability in meta-analysis. *Educational Researcher* 1982, June-July: 10-14. [Qual]

Strinivasan C, Zhou M. A note on pooling Kaplan-Meier estimates. *Biometrics* 1993; 49: 861–4. [M-A]

Sugita M, Kanamori M, Izuno T, Miyakawa M. Estimating a

summarized odds ratio whilst eliminating publication bias in meta-analysis. *Japanese Journal of Clinical Oncology* 1992; **22**: 354–8. [Id]

Thacker SB. Meta-analysis: a quantitative approach to research integration. *JAMA* 1988; **259**: 1685–9. [Gen]

Thompson SG. Why sources of heterogeneity in meta-analysis should be investigated. *BMJ* 1994; **309**: 1351–5. [M-A]

Thompson SG, Pocock SJ. Can meta-analyses be trusted? *Lancet* 1991; **338**: 1127–30. [M-A]

Vandenbroucke JP. Passive smoking and lung cancer: a publication bias? *BMJ* 1988; **296**: 391–2. [Id]

Vanderkerchove P, O'Donovan PA, Lilford RJ, Harada TW. Infertility treatment: from cookery to science. The epidemiology of randomised controlled trials. *Br J Obstet Gynaecol* 1993; **100**: 1005–36. [Id]

Van der Wijden CL, Overbeke AJPM. Gerandomiseerde klinische trials in het *Nederlands Tijdschrift voor Geneeskund*. *Ned Tijdschr Geneeskd* 1993; **137**: 1607–10. [Id]

Van Houwelingen HC, Zwinderman KH, Stijnen T. A bivariate approach to meta-analysis. *Stat Med* 1993; **12**: 2273–84. [M-A]

Veldhuyzen van Zanten SJO, Boers M. Metanalyse: de kunst van het systematisch oversicht. *Ned Tijdschr Geneeskd* 1993; **137**: 1594–9. [Gen]

Walker AM, Martin-Moreno JM, Artalejo FR. Odd man out: a graphical approach to meta-analysis. *Am J Pub Health* 1988; **78**: 961–6. [M-A, Rep]

West RR. A look at the statistical overview (or meta-analysis). *J R Coll Phys Lond* 1993; **27**: 111–5. [M-A]

Whitehead A, Whitehead J. A general parametric approach to the meta-analysis of randomized clinical trials. *Stat Med* 1991; **10**: 1665–77. [M-A]

Williams DH, Davis CE. Reporting on assignment methods in clinical trials. *Controlled Clin Trials* 1994; **15**: 294–8. [Qual]

Yates F, Cochran WG. The analysis of groups of experiments. *Journal of Agricultural Sciences* 1938; **28**: 556–80. [M-A]

Yusuf S, Peto R, Lewis J, Collins R, Sleight P. Beta blockade during and after myocardial infarction: an overview of the randomized trials. *Prog Cardiovasc Dis* 1985; **27**: 335–71. [M-A]

Yusuf S, Wittes J, Probstfield J, Tyroler HA. Analysis and interpretation of treatment effects in subgroups of patients in randomized clinical trials. *JAMA* 1991; **266**: 93–8. [Rep]

# Index

# Related titles

## HOW TO WRITE A PAPER

*Edited by G M Hall*

This short book provides all the practical information on how to get a paper accepted. It has chapters on each section of a scientific paper from Introduction to Discussion. With contributions from editors of international journals including the *BMJ*, *British Journal of Anaesthesia*, and *Cardiovascular Research*, it explains in a refreshingly direct way what journal editors are looking for in a good paper.

Readership: all medical professionals, scientific researchers

ISBN 0 7279 0822 7   128 pages   1994

## *By the same author*
## STATISTICS IN PRACTICE

*Sheila M Gore, Douglas G Altman*

This important and authoritative book explains how to design studies, apply statistical techniques, and interpret studies using statistics. It is presented simply enough to be understood by those with no statistical training.

Readership: doctors, nurses, therapists, students

ISBN 0 7279 0085 4   107 pages   1982

118

# STATISTICS WITH CONFIDENCE

*Martin J Gardner, Douglas G Altman*

An essential guide for everyone using statistical methods to present their findings, this book gives the reasons for using confidence intervals, followed by detailed methods of calculation, including numerous worked examples and especially compiled tables.

"The great value of this book is that it presents in an easily understood form, the methods which will be needed in most situations." *Journal of Epidemiology and Community Health*

Readership: students, medical researchers, doctors

ISBN 0 7279 0222 9   156 pages   1989

For further details of these books and our full range of titles write to Marketing Department, BMJ Publishing Group, BMA House, Tavistock Square, London WC1H 9JR or telephone Diana Chapple on 0171 383 6541.